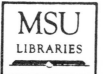

Atlas of Lymph Node Pathology

To
Emma Louise,
James
and
Ben

Current Histopathology

Consultant Editor
Professor G. Austin Gresham, TD, ScD, MD, FRC Path.
Professor of Morbid Anatomy and Histology, University of Cambridge

Volume One

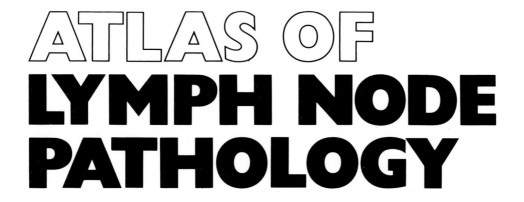

ATLAS OF LYMPH NODE PATHOLOGY

BY JEANNE ARNO

Department of Pathology
University of Cambridge

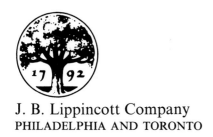

J. B. Lippincott Company
PHILADELPHIA AND TORONTO

Published and distributed in North America by
J. B. Lippincott Company

Published in Great Britain by
MTP Press Limited
Falcon House, Cable Street
Lancaster, England

ISBN 0—397—50451—9

LCCN 79—89970

Printed in Great Britain

Contents

Current Histopathology Series

Consultant Editor's Note

At the present time books on morbid anatomy and histology can be divided into two broad groups: extensive textbooks often written primarily for students and monographs on research topics.

This takes no account of the fact that the vast majority of pathologists are involved in an essentially practical field of general Diagnostic Pathology, providing an important service to their clinical colleagues. Many of these pathologists are expected to cover a broad range of disciplines and even those who remain solely within the field of histopathology usually have single and sole responsibility within the hospital for all this work. They may often have no chance for direct discussion on problem cases with colleagues in the same department. In the field of histopathology, no less than in other medical fields, there have been extensive and recent advances, not only in new histochemical techniques but also in the type of specimen provided by new surgical procedures.

There is a great need for the provision of appropriate information for this group. This need has been defined in the following terms.

1. It should be aimed at the general clinical pathologist or histopathologist with existing practical training, but should also have value for the trainee pathologist.

2. It should concentrate on the practical aspects of histopathology taking account of the new techniques which should be within the compass of the worker in a unit with reasonable facilities.
3. New types of material e.g. those derived from endoscopic biopsy should be covered fully.
4. There should be an adequate number of illustrations on each subject to demonstrate the variation in appearance that is encountered.
5. Colour illustrations should be used wherever they aid recognition.

The present concept stemmed from this definition but it was immediately realized that these aims could only be achieved within the compass of a series, of which this volume is one. Since histopathology is, by its very nature, systematized, the individual volumes deal with one system or where this appears more appropriate with a single organ.

In selecting authors for the volumes I have deliberately concentrated on those who are not only experts in the field but also have an adequate breadth of experience in the problems of current diagnostic histopathology. This should ensure the practical approach that is the keynote of the series and guarantee that the books are used constantly on the workbench and not relegated to the library shelf.

G. Austin Gresham
Cambridge

Introduction

The scope of this book includes several controversial areas and it is impossible to give an account which satisfies everyone, including the author. However, the prime objective has been to aid in the interpretation of histopathological appearances in lymph nodes. To that end, there is some attempt at rationalization whilst admitting that, in rationalizing biological processes, there is a danger of distortion and inconsistency.

Normal structure and function of lymph nodes is taken as the backbone from which reactive changes on the one hand, and neoplastic transformation on the other, can be seen to take their origin. Where the backbone itself is faulty, then there occur disturbances of immunological function, which engender another group of histological changes. Lastly, essentially systemic disorders may be reflected in lymph nodes.

This simple approach can be used to bring order to an apparent chaos of histological appearances and pathological processes. It is capable of sophistication to match breadth of knowledge. No doubt some concepts expressed in this book already require modification, since new insights are reported constantly in this field of study. Such apparent instability of viewpoint and nomenclature has made many wary, but it is hoped that an underlying simple basis will allow future changes to be easily assimilated.

Detailed accounts of methods of classification are omitted, being widely available elsewhere, nor is there any attempt to be comprehensive. The discussion is limited almost exclusively to the appearances in routine sections, stained with haematoxylin and eosin, with the addition of a few special stains, since additional technical methods are not always available. The limitations that this imposes are acknowledged.

Acknowledgements
I should like to thank:
Mrs Mary Wright who typed the manuscript; the Technical Staff of the Histology Laboratory, Addenbrooke's Hospital for the preparation of many extra sections; the Staff of the Department of Medical Photography and Illustration, Addenbrooke's Hospital for their facilites and advice; and above all, the people who provided the time for me to write, my colleagues in histopathology.

Techniques

Lymph node biopsy is performed when there is unexplained enlargement of one or more nodes. The surgeon should be encouraged to remove the largest node where possible, even if it is not the most easily accessible, since it can be expected to show the most advanced changes. Smaller, more superficial nodes, whilst obviously abnormal, may not provide adequate diagnostic material. The other essential is that the node should be excised whole, since the interpretation of fragments is quite unreliable and distortion of the tissue prior to fixation must be avoided.

The subsequent handling of the biopsied node varies with local pathological resources. In some centres, fresh cell suspensions are prepared for subsequent surface marker studies and cell culture. Imprint preparations can be made from the cut surfaces of the fresh tissue for cytochemical investigation. In most cases these are air-dried, and fixed later, but a few may be fixed immediately, whilst still wet, as is done with other cytological preparations.

Whilst it is important to process the tissue used to make the imprints, for histological examination, so that both techniques can be compared, often the 'dabbing' process causes distortion and in any case delays fixation. It is therefore essential to remove tissue for histological examination first, and place it in fixative. At the same time, if electron microscopy is available, then a small amount of the tissue should be suitably prepared.

For routine histological examination, fixation in an adequate volume of 10% neutral buffered formal–saline is preferred. Whole nodes or large pieces should be cut transversely with a very sharp blade to allow penetration of fixative. Fixation should last about 24 hours in all; unduly long periods of fixation are not desirable and may interfere with subsequent staining. Although sections of a thickness in general use for surgical histology (about 5 μm)

may be adequate, it is often necessary, especially in densely cellular tissue, to request thin sections (2 μm), as it may be impossible to appreciate the cytology of individual cells. Indeed an extremely elegant method of histological examination, used extensively in some centres for study of lymph nodes, is the use of very thin sections (1 μm), achieved by embedding the tissue in methacrylate. The necessity of a really sharp knife edge for section cutting, no matter which technique is in use, cannot be over-emphasized. At low power, scores across the field can make interpretation difficult, and at high power, individual cells are damaged beyond recognition.

Routinely, sections are stained with haematoxylin and eosin (H & E) and some form of silver impregnation method to demonstrate the reticulin fibre framework should be done in addition. Also used frequently in the study of lymph nodes are pyronin and methyl green (PMG) and periodic acid Schiff (PAS) staining methods. In certain cases, it is useful to demonstrate the presence of neutrophil leukocytes in paraffin sections by Leder's naphthol AS–D chloroacetate esterase method[1].

Another technique for examining sections of formal–saline fixed tissue prepared from routine paraffin-wax blocks, is the immuno-peroxidase method (Figure 2.8), which is being increasingly widely applied in different fields of study. It has been used to identify cell populations in lymphomas, and is perhaps most helpful where a B cell proliferation of uncertain nature can be demonstrated to be monoclonal in type.

References

1. Leder, L. D. (1964). The selective enzymocytochemical demonstration of neutrophil myeloid cells and tissue mast cells in paraffin sections. *Klin. Wochenschr.*, **42**, 553.

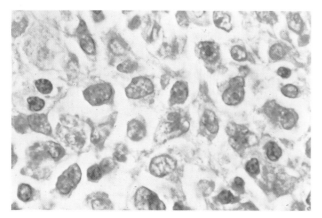

Figure 2.1 A large cell lymphoma similar in type of that shown in Figure 2.2. Poor fixation results in shrinkage of the cytoplasm and obscuring of nuclear detail. H & E ×910.

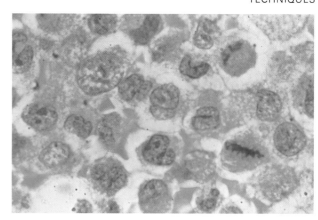

Figure 2.2 Even here, fixation of every single cell is not ideal, but nuclear and cytoplasmic features are better demonstrated. H & E ×910.

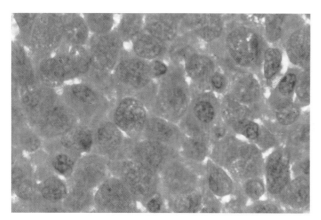

Figure 2.3 A thick section, in which, despite adequate fixation, cellular detail is obscured. H & E ×910.

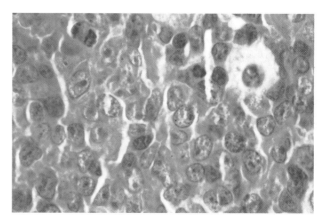

Figure 2.4 Splitting artefacts caused by cutting the section with a blunt knife. H & E ×910.

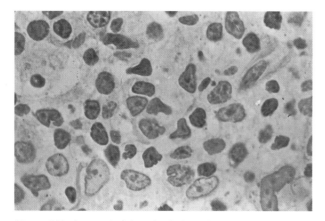

Figure 2.5 Improved nuclear detail shown in a thin section (1 μm); the field includes small cleaved follicular centre cells. H & E ×910.

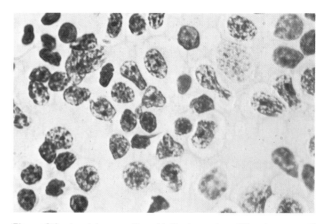

Figure 2.6 Imprint preparation of follicular centre cell lymphoma, small cleaved cell type. Cytofix applied to smear before drying. Giemsa ×910.

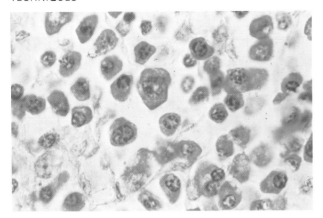

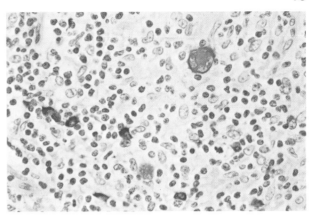

Figure 2.7 Pyronin positivity of cytoplasm of plasma cells and nucleoli. Pyronin methyl green ×910.

Figure 2.8 Immunoperoxidase reaction. Positive brown staining of some plasma cells and a Reed–Sternberg cell, following application of antibody to IgG to a section from a case of Hodgkin's disease. Haematoxylin ×365.

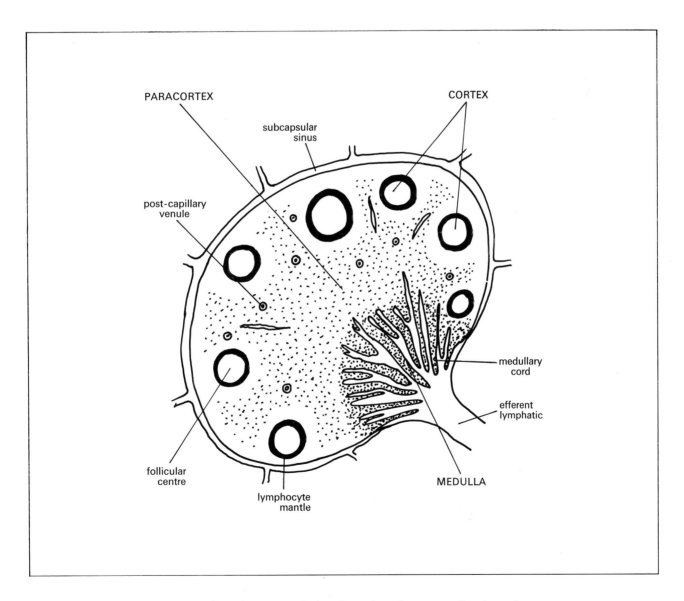

Plate I Diagram of the functional areas of a lymph node.

Unlike most other tissues, the generally held concept of a lymph node does not represent the inevitable result of spontaneous maturation of lymphoid tissue. Rather, at any given stage, it reflects the response to those stimuli affecting it.

Lymph nodes have evolved as sites of interaction, where both circulating and sedentary cells are brought into intimate contact with each other, and also with stimuli carried either by the draining lymph or the blood stream. In normal circumstances, the lymph nodes in the new-born are present as delicate reticulin frameworks, populated by small numbers of lymphocytes which aggregate in the cortical areas.

The underlying architecture can be clearly appreciated at this stage of development (Figure 3.1). Afferent lymphatic channels empty into the marginal or peripheral sinus, beneath the capsule. At the inner surface of the marginal sinus commences the richer reticulin network of the node pulp, in which the lymphocyte aggregations occur, and through which lymph percolates, passing through fine sinusoids. When it reaches the medulla of the node, larger sinuses collect the lymph and channel it towards the efferent lymphatic vessel which leaves the hilum. Separating the medullary sinuses are elongated structures formed of reticulin fibres and destined to be populated by lymphoid cells, often showing differentiation towards plasma cells. These structures are the medullary cords.

The system of sinuses, through which the draining lymph passes, is lined by large cells of histiocyte/macrophage type. Sometimes these cells appear to be attached to the wall by only one or two fine processes, and dangle in the lumen, providing a refined, sieve-like function (Figure 3.12).

Cortex and Medulla

In the outer region of the node pulp, destined to form the definitive cortex, there are other specialized cells, the dendritic reticular cells. Their nuclei are slightly irregular with a delicate peripheral rim of chromatin and a small distinct nucleolus. They are characterized by long, fine cytoplasmic processes which are insinuated between the adjacent cells, a feature which can be seen clearly in ultra-thin sections. Electron microscopy also demonstrates that these dendritic processes of separate cells are bound to each other by desmosome junctions.

Much of the antigenic material reaching a lymph node is brought in the afferent lymph. The detailed handling of such material has been found to depend on its physical state, ease of breakdown and whether or not it is linked to any pre-existing antibody (which greatly enhances the uptake). In essence, however, the system of macrophages within the sinuses acts as a living, phagocytic filter as lymph drains slowly through the node. Some of the antigen taken up by the sinus macrophages can be shown subsequently on the surface of the processes of the dendritic reticular cells, this localization being dependent on the presence of the C3 component of complement.

The antigen-bearing dendritic cells tend to aggregate (Figure 3.3) and, in close association with them, lymphocyte transformation occurs, so that larger cells with vesicular nuclei, distinct nucleoli and abundant pyroninophilic cytoplasm are seen. Mitotic figures occur and may be frequent. Therefore, in the middle of the rather ill-defined collections of small lymphocytes of the cortex, the primary follicles, there now appear paler areas, pale by virtue of the fact that they contain cells with less dense nuclei and more cytoplasm than the surrounding lymphocytes. These pale areas, which tend to be round in outline, are the germinal or follicular centres (Figure 3.5).

During phases of activity, follicular centres have a very pleomorphic appearance. Macrophages containing remnants of nuclear material may be numerous. It appears that much of the proliferative activity which occurs results in the production of cells which are in some way unsuitable, and they are destroyed within the follicular centre itself. Dendritic reticular cells, of course, form part of the population, as do a small number of plasma cells. The majority of cells however are lymphoid in type, but their cytological appearance is very variable and this aspect is mentioned again in the section dealing with follicular lymphomas (pages 67–70).

From observations of the mixture of lymphoid cells, certain generalizations have been made. Some of the cells have extremely irregular nuclei, often with deep notches in their outline, or folds appearing as heavy lines. Some of these notched nuclei are only a little larger than those of normal small lymphocytes, but others are considerably larger. It's usually difficult to distinguish their cytoplasm. The presence of the deep indentations has led to the designation 'cleaved' cells, in contradistinction to which are the 'non-cleaved' lymphoid cells of the follicular centres, with large oval to round open nuclei and distinct nucleoli. This variable cytological appearance, together with considerable mitotic activity, can cause a normal reactive follicular centre to resemble a highly malignant tumour, when viewed at high power (Figure 3.7). Most of the lymphoid cells found in the follicular centres have been shown to be B lymphocytes. Virgin B cells leave the bone marrow to circulate in the bloodstream which they leave by adhering to, and then squeezing between, the specialized tall, endo-

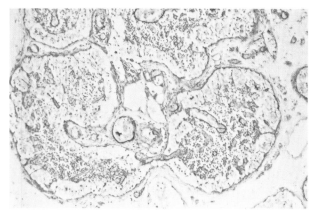

Figure 3.1 A lymph node from a week-old infant. The delicate framework with a well marked subcapsular sinus and scanty cellular population is shown in a reticulin stained section. Reticulin ×91.

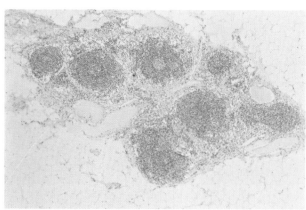

Figure 3.2 Subsequent development of nodal tissue. Lymphoid aggregates with central, paler follicular centres appear. H & E ×36.5.

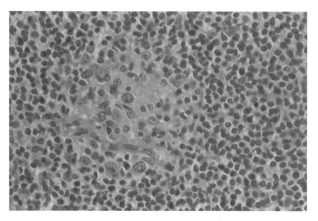

Figure 3.3 An early stage in the formation of a follicular centre. Larger cells with eosinophilic cytoplasm, some at least being dendritic reticular cells, accumulate in the vicinity of a small blood vessel. H & E ×365.

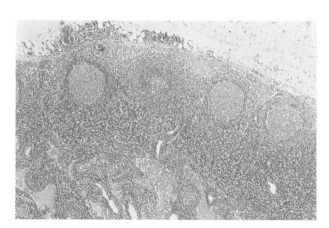

Figure 3.4 All the functional zones of a reactive lymph node are demonstrated here, with follicles in the outer cortex, faintly mottled paracortex and medulla with widely dilated sinuses. H & E ×36.5.

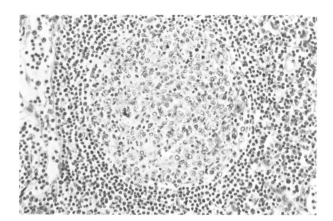

Figure 3.5 A follicular centre. Its pallor is due to the fact that it is composed of larger cells and the neat concentric rings of the lymphocyte mantle give it sharp definition. H & E ×91.

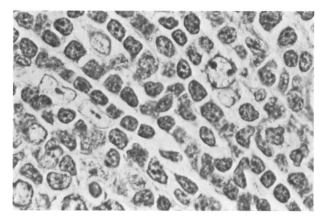

Figure 3.6 Lymphocyte mantle. The edge of a follicular centre is present in the lower right-hand corner. The surrounding small lymphocytes have a regimented appearance. Phosphotungstic acid haematoxylin (PTAH) ×910.

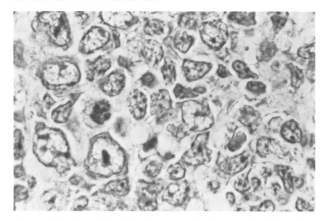

Figure 3.7 A reactive follicular centre showing considerable nuclear pleomorphism. Small cleaved cells and large non-cleaved cells are easily distinguished. Often the nucleoli in the latter are seen close to the nuclear membrane. PTAH ×910.

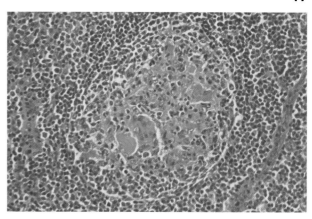

Figure 3.8 A small follicular centre with PAS positive material accumulating within it. This can progress to a 'burnt-out' appearance with very few cells remaining. H & E ×91.

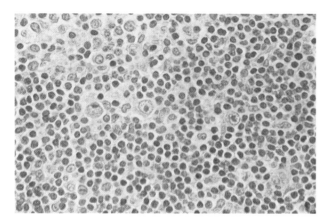

Figure 3.9 Paracortical area populated by small lymphocytes and transformed lymphocytes, often with large nucleoli which tend to be centrally placed. H & E ×365.

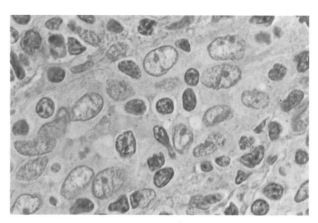

Figure 3.10 A post-capillary venule with lymphocytes migrating outwards through the wall, shown well in a thin section. H & E ×910.

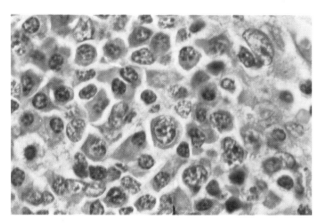

Figure 3.11 Area of B lymphocyte proliferation with production of mature plasma cells in a reactive node. H & E ×910.

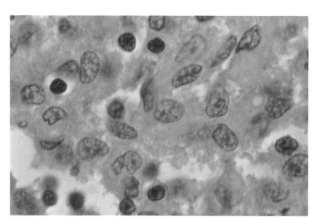

Figure 3.12 Histiocytes within a sinus in a reactive node. H & E ×910.

thelial cells of post-capillary venules, situated in the interfollicular areas of lymphoid tissues. They then migrate, responding to some unknown stimulus, to the cortical areas and apparently pass into the follicular centres to undergo a phase of antigen-driven proliferative activity.

Clearly, there is opportunity for intimate contact with antigens in a refined micro-environment and presumably the unusual morphological changes associated with this proliferative phase of development has functional significance. It is assumed, but not proved, that the B cells emerging from the follicular centres are memory cells, committed to production of a clone of secretory plasma cells when further suitable antigenic stimulation occurs. Conceivably, for a few of them this may take place in the node in which they originate, during their passage through the thymus-dependent area, where they come into intimate contact with T lymphocytes, and they may then come to populate the medullary cords. From there, their secreted immunoglobulin can pass directly into the lymph leaving the node.

The majority of the memory B cells however, drain away in the efferent lymph to enter the blood stream and then migrate across specialized endothelial sites to pass through other thymus-independent areas of lymphoid tissue.

Paracortex

The interfollicular area of the unstimulated lymph node is quite ill-defined, populated by small lymphocytes but lacking the characteristic follicles of the cortex. It can expand however to form a definite functional zone, the paracortex, as a result of stimulation. Its flexibility results from the fact that it is merely the site through which circulating T cells pass, unless appropriate stimulation causes their arrest and subsequent proliferation. It may then become conspicuous, with the increase in its cell population compressing, even almost obliterating the cortex, or at least separating it from the medullary zone.

At times of paracortical activity, numerous large transformed lymphocytes can give a spotty appearance against the background of small lymphocytes, and mitoses may be numerous. The picture may be further modified by the presence of histiocytes in the area, as discussed under reactive changes.

Traffic of Lymphocytes through Lymph Nodes

Reference has already been made to the route taken by B lymphocytes of bone marrow origin to reach the follicular centres. However, other B lymphocytes, which have been produced in follicular centres elsewhere, then cross the post-capillary venule endothelium in like manner (Figure 3.10) and also migrate out towards the cortex, where they move through the zone immediately adjacent to the follicular centres. They do not apparently enter the latter, but then move slowly towards the medulla across the paracortex. The stimuli controlling this migratory pathway are unknown.

Techniques employing injected labelled T and B lymphocytes[1] have given rough estimates for the time this intra-nodal passage takes and in the case of B lymphocytes it is from 30 to 36 hours.

The T lymphocytes also cross the venule endothelium but their migratory route is more direct since they take, as it were, the line of least resistance and move through the interfollicular area towards the medullary sinuses, taking some 16–18 hours in transit.

Regression and Atrophy

Besides forming and enlarging, follicular centres can regress. Especially in older age groups they may be scanty, small in size and lacking mitotic activity. The dendritic reticular cells may appear more prominent under these conditions. Eosinophilic, PAS-positive material often appears as a deposit in follicular centres (Figure 3.8) (it is frequent in the spleen) and probably represent a mixture of components. Sometimes it remains, in the wake of lymphoid cells which have disappeared, and the impression is then one of a 'burnt-out' centre.

In advanced atrophy, nodes lose much of their cell population altogether, and this is accompanied by loss of the reticulin scaffolding to some extent, with replacement of the central area by adipose tissue. Often, the nodes in a mastectomy specimen from a middle-aged woman consist only of a thin rim of lymphoid tissue beneath the capsule, surrounding the adipose centre. However, under the influence of renewed stimulation, this central area can be repopulated.

References

1. Ford, W. L. (1975). Lymphocyte migration and immune responses. *Prog. Allergy*, **19**, 1–48.

Introduction

Out of an understanding of the function and organization of lymph nodes, the possible response patterns emerge. Clear cut responses are usually seen only under experimental conditions, and in practice we are most frequently looking at a mixture of effects. However some basic theoretical concepts aid analysis in any given case. The account given here considers each of the elements in turn.

The Cortex: Follicular Hyperplasia

Where the stimulus promotes mainly B cell proliferation, there is an increase in the size and number of follicular centres, and of the activity within them (Figure 4.1). The corollary of this increased production of B cells, is that the end-product, the plasma cells, become numerous and are especially noticeable in the medullary cords. They are however also present in the interfollicular areas. The well-defined follicular centres, with their surrounding coronas of small lymphocytes, may take over most of the node, almost obliterating the paracortex and invading the medulla. Usually these reactive centres are round in shape and this is reflected in any cross section through them, but sometimes they can be greatly elongated, or 'waisted' in outline (Figure 5.5). When they include active macrophages the presence of these scattered cells, with their abundant pale staining cytoplasm, gives an appearance of holes in the otherwise densely cellular area and this is frequently referred to as a 'starry sky' appearance.

The Paracortex

The changes which affect this area of a lymph node are far more complex. It is helpful to consider it from two aspects, although admittedly the distinction is an artificial one. Firstly an 'active' response by T cells which are held, stimulated and proliferate (Figure 4.3), as a result of appropriate antigenic stimulation. In some cases the picture can evolve further, with the addition of histiocytes. The histiocytes then undergo morphological changes (epithelioid cells) and become organized into defined clusters (granulomas) (Figure 4.4), probably under the influence of T cells.

Secondly, there may be a 'passive' expansion of the paracortical area, in which the number of histiocytes present is greatly increased (Figure 4.6). Drainage from the periphery may be a contributory factor in this. The accumulation of cells is related to the presence of materials within their cytoplasm, either products of metabolism or even micro-organisms. Histiocytes may also be increased in the lymphocyte-depleted paracortex of immunodeficiency disorders.

The Sinuses

These become a conspicuous feature either if they are dilated, with abundant lymph flow through them, as is the normal appearance in mesenteric nodes, or if their cell content is increased. This may be accompanied by evidence of ingested material, especially if it is pigmented or not readily broken down. In some cases it may elicit a granulomatous response from the sinus histiocytes, especially a 'foreign body' reaction. Where many cells accumulate in the sinuses, then they may spill over and expand the paracortical area.

Another important cause of sinus prominence can be the presence of other cell types within the spaces, haematopoietic cells or neoplastic cells for example.

Other Reactive Features

Acute Inflammation

In acutely inflamed lymph nodes, the changes are akin to those seen in other tissues, with vasodilatation, infiltration by neutrophil leukocytes and possibly areas of necrosis. Usually these non-specific changes are accompanied by those specific to the lymphoid tissue, with responses in the lymphoid cells, evidenced by mitotic activity and cell transformation.

Chronic Inflammation

There is often fibrous thickening of the capsule and this may be infiltrated by cells, especially lymphocytes, which stray out into the surrounding tissues. Gradually, fibrous scarring can come to replace areas of the node itself.

Blood Vessel Changes

The post-capillary venules may become much more obvious, because of increase in size of the endothelial cells. These seem taller than usual with enlarged, plump nuclei and many lymphocytes are emigrating between them. Other changes to be noted are necrosis of vessel walls, cuffing by plasma cells, or deposition of amyloid.

Sometimes the interfollicular area appears expanded and this is due to an apparent proliferation of blood vessels, between which can occur a rather mixed cellular population, although plasma cells are usually much in evidence.

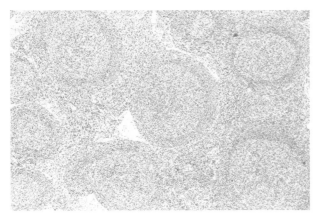

Figure 4.1 Follicular hyperplasia from a case of rheumatoid arthritis. In this example large, approximately round follicular centres surrounded by wide lymphocyte mantles dominate the histological appearance. H & E ×36.5.

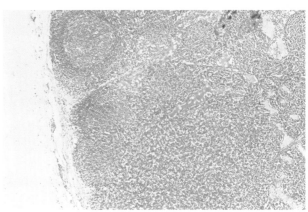

Figure 4.2 Active paracortical response. Much of the nodal tissue shown here consists of expanded paracortex of a 'starry' pattern. There is however some follicular response at the same time. H & E ×36.5

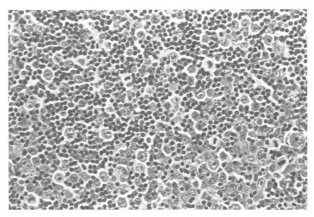

Figure 4.3 Active paracortical response. The 'starry' appearance is seen to be due to the presence of numerous immunoblasts against a background of small lymphocytes. H & E ×230.

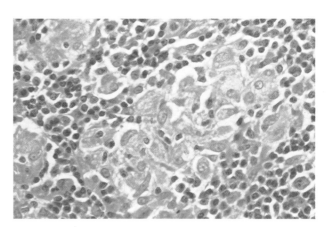

Figure 4.4 Epithelioid histiocytes. Clusters of these cells contribute to a granulomatous response. H & E ×365.

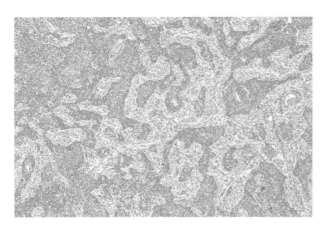

Figure 4.5 Sinus hyperplasia. The sinuses in this node are widely dilated but are populated by numerous histiocytes whose abundant cytoplasm gives a pale eosinophilic appearance. H & E ×36.5.

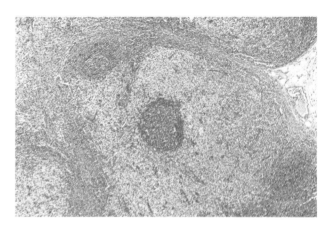

Figure 4.6 Passive paracortical expansion. A lymph node showing only residual follicular structures. The paracortex contributes the bulk of the tissue and has a pale, somewhat uniform appearance, due to accumulation of histiocytes. An example of dermatopathic lymphadenopathy. H & E ×36.5.

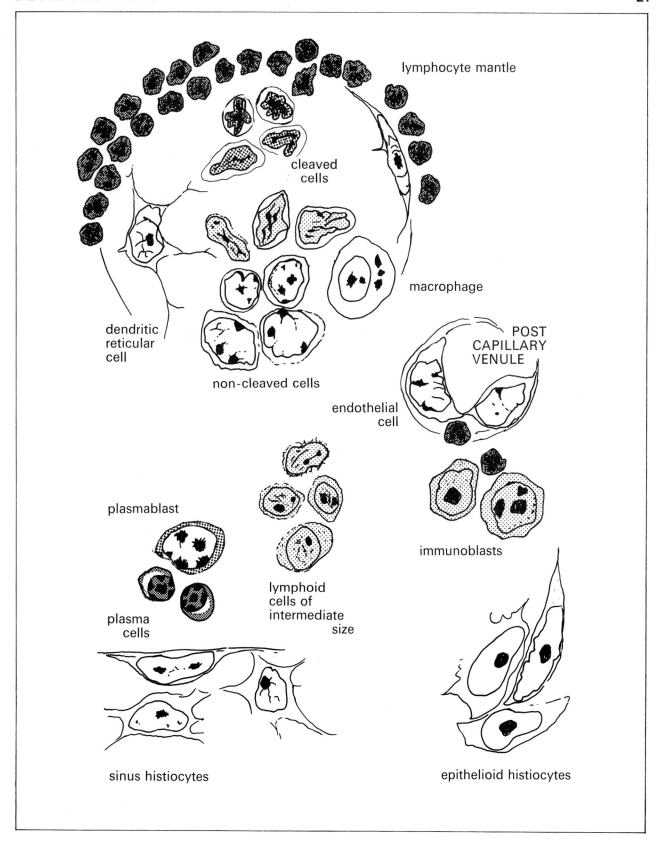

Plate II   Diagram to illustrate some cell types found in
reactive lymph nodes.

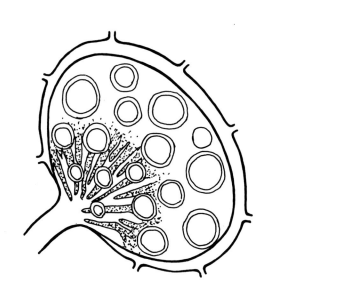

1 Follicular hyperplasia

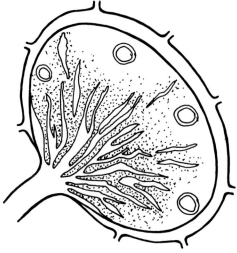

2 Sinus hyperplasia

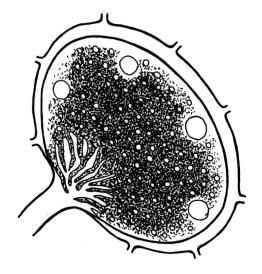

3 'Active' paracortical response

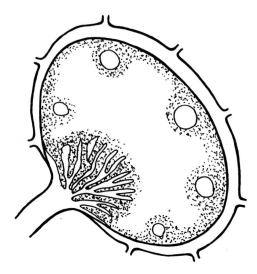

4 'Passive' paracortical expansion

Plate III   Basic reactive patterns in lymph nodes.

Follicular Hyperplasia

Introduction

The presence of lymphoid follicles with follicular or germinal centres simply reflects normal activity in a lymph node, and in most cases some are present. It is only appropriate to use the term 'follicular hyperplasia' where increase in their size and number contribute to significant lymph node enlargement. In the majority of instances this is encountered in association with other reactive changes, the exception being rheumatoid arthritis.

Rheumatoid Arthritis

A massive and overwhelming follicular response can occur in phases of activity in this condition. Rarely, the lymph node enlargement can dominate the clinical picture and lead to the erroneous impression that the patient has a lymphoma, since the joint symptoms are quite overshadowed. Such a node, being submitted with the brief clinical information '? lymphoma', can easily be misinterpreted as a follicular lymphoma by the pathologist. This is because when examined at low power, the entire node appears to have been taken over by follicular structures; a more careful evaluation reveals that the architecture is not in fact destroyed, and that although follicles appear in the medullary region, they simply expand pre-existing cords, and the sinuses persist as before.

Moreover, the follicular centres exhibit the pleomorphic appearance of activity, with numerous mitoses, some plasma cells and usually abundant phagocytic macrophages. Further evidence of this being normal activity is provided by the enormous number of mature plasma cells which such a node contains, both in the interfollicular zones, and the medullary cords. Amongst them Russell bodies may be found.

There are other pointers to reactivity, with increase in the size of the endothelial cells of post-capillary venules, and in the sinuses the histiocytes are large, showing evidence of phagocytosis. There are often some neutrophils present also.

In the small percentage of cases of rheumatoid arthritis which exhibit amyloid in the blood vessel walls of other tissues, this may also be identified within the lymph nodes[1].

Childhood and Adolescence

During the early stages of normal development, there is continual exposure of cells of the immune system to antigenic stimuli. One of the commonest findings in examining lymph nodes from children is that the enlargement is due predominantly to follicular hyperplasia. As often as not, the finding is quite non-specific, in fact no other significant change can be recognized. Presumably the few nodes which come to be examined in this way, merely represent the tip of the normal 'iceberg', and are only excised at all because they persist a little longer than usual, or are even noticed.

Giant Follicular Hyperplasia

Sometimes excised lymph nodes show this very characteristic form of reactive change. The follicular centres are much larger than those normally encountered, often being enormously elongated, and frequently dumb-bell shaped, or even more bizarre in outline (Figure 5.5). Phagocytic macrophages are prominent throughout these extraordinary structures (Figure 5.3). The cause of this particular change is as yet unknown but presumably is infective. A cluster of three such cases occurred within a few months of each other in this area two or three years ago. The enlarged nodes eventually subside, after several months.

Large follicular centres with bizarre outlines are also encountered as a part of the other changes in toxoplasmosis and, to some extent in syphilis.

Measles

Measles is included in this section because the follicular hyperplasia which forms part of the histological appearance is particularly eye-catching, due to the presence of the enormous Warthin-Finkeldey giant cells which occur, both within the follicular centres and immediately adjacent to them. These multinucleated cells can contain as many as a hundred nuclei, each a little larger and less dense than that of a normal small lymphocyte. They have a distinct chromatin network and it may be possible to find small nucleoli within them. Many of these nuclei however are found to be undergoing pyknosis and degeneration and they may then be phagocytosed by large, and also multinucleated, macrophages within the follicular centres. The sinuses too contain multinucleated histiocytes (Figure 5.7). Other changes are non-specific in nature, with an overall increase in enlarged lymphoid cells and some apparent proliferation of small blood vessels.

The characteristic appearance of the lymphoid tissues in this virus infection is seen rarely. It is present during the prodromal stage for about a week before the appearance of the rash, and disappears soon afterwards. It is most likely to be encountered in the tonsils or vermiform appendix, but may present in a lymph node biopsy, especially following measles vaccination[2].

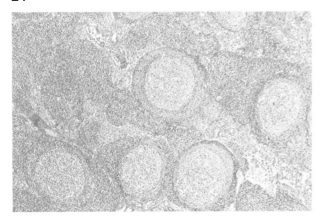

Figure 5.1 Rheumatoid arthritis. The proliferation of lymphoid follicles with active follicular centres may come to dominate the entire node. H & E   × 36.5.

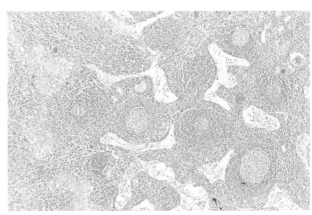

Figure 5.2 Follicular hyperplasia. Lymphoid follicles invade the medullary cords. H & E   × 36.5.

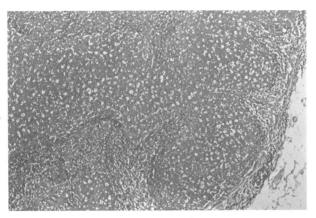

Figure 5.3 Follicular hyperplasia characterized by greatly enlarged follicular centres, with a conspicuous 'starry sky' appearance can cause confusion with lymphomas of Burkitt-type, particularly if the node is fragmented during removal. H & E   × 36.5.

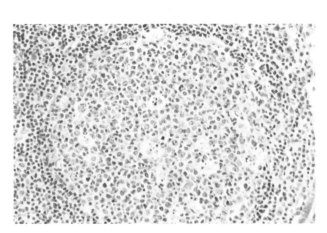

Figure 5.4 The 'starry sky' appearance is caused by scattered large macrophages within the follicular centres. This is seen commonly in childhood. H & E   × 230.

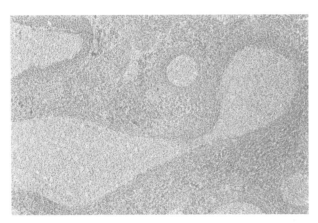

Figure 5.5 Forms of predominantly follicular hyperplasia occur, which are characterized by unusually large follicular centres, often bizarre in outline. H & E   × 36.5.

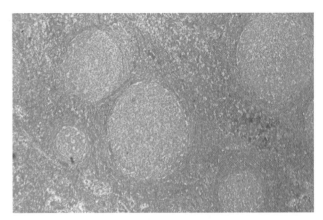

Figure 5.6 The follicular structures seen throughout the node in this case showed some cytological variation but largely lacked lymphocytic mantles. The question of early follicular lymphoma was raised, but the interfollicular tissue showed normal reactive changes, and the patient is well four years later. H & E   × 36.5.

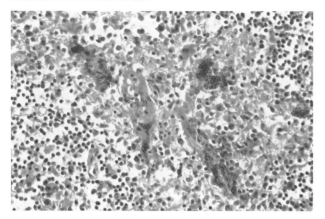

Figure 5.7 Measles. The formation of enormous multinucleated cells is characteristic of infection by this virus. In this particular node, obtained at necropsy examination, such cells were still present, but only apparently within sinuses. H & E ×91.

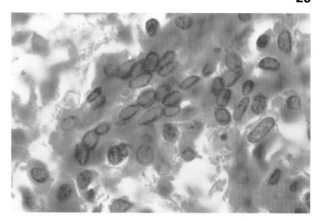

Figure 5.8 Multinucleated cell within a sinus in measles infection. H & E ×365.

References

1. Nosanchuk, J. S. and Schnitzer, B. (1969). Follicular hyperplasia in lymph nodes from patients with rheumatoid arthritis. *Cancer*, **24**, 343.

2. Shannon Allen, M. Jr., Talbot, W. H. and McDonald, R. M. (1966). Atypical lymph node hyperplasia after administration of attenuated, live measles vaccine. *N. Engl. J. Med.*, **274**, 677.

Introduction

The 'active' response may be dominated by changes in the lymphocyte population, with recruitment, mitotic activity and transformation. This is particularly seen in response to certain virus infections in the early stages, and also in lymph nodes draining the area of a homograft, or of skin exhibiting contact hypersensitivity.

On low-power examination, the expanded paracortex appears spotty, due to the large number of transformed lymphocytes, and on detailed examination the appearance can be mistaken for a highly malignant neoplasm, because of the mitotic rate, and large lymphoid cells which are present in the sinuses. However careful evaluation shows that although the process is so florid, it is not purposeless, and confines itself to the paracortex, without destructive effects on the rest of the node.

Usually in association with a longer time course, but also depending upon the stimulus, histiocytes can appear in the same area and may be sufficient to impart a paler appearance. Often they are in loose clusters or may be organized into more clearly defined granulomas. This behaviour indicates that they are responding to the influence of the stimulated T lymphocytes, and is the histological expression of immunological cellular response to certain antigens.

Particular patterns of granulomatous reaction are usually indicative to some extent of the agent which is initiating them. However, since a granuloma only represents host response and is governed by T lymphocyte activity, it is not an invariable finding in association with a specific stimulus. Pathologists trained in Europe have a clear concept of what is to be expected in tuberculous inflammation for example, but the same agent, *Mycobacterium tuberculosis*, can produce a very different response in some individuals, particularly if encountered in non-European hosts.

However, in many cases the pattern of a particular granuloma is a good guide to the causative agent, animate or inanimate, and enables the cause to be sought. Only a few of the many granulomatous conditions which can affect lymph nodes are referred to here. Symmers[1] gives a wide-ranging account of conditions causing chronic lymphadenitis including many of the more unusual examples of granulomatous inflammation.

Vaccinia

A lucid description of the changes in lymph nodes draining an area of vaccination is given by Hartsock[2]. In the first four days, the changes include necrosis of blood vessels with inflammation and oedema of the capsule, but thereafter there are combinations of paracortical and follicular responses. At about eight days after inoculation, the dominant change is expansion of the paracortex, which exhibits a strikingly mottled appearance, with numerous transformed lymphocytes. At this stage, the virus can be cultured from the nodal tissue.

About a week later, follicular hyperplasia and plasma cell infiltrates become more apparent. At all stages, eosinophil leukocytes in varying numbers can be present. This fact, together with the presence of many mitoses and large, sometimes polyploid, transformed cells with conspicuous nucleoli, has led at times to a confusion with Hodgkin's disease, because strangely enough the history of vaccination is discounted or overlooked. However, as Dorfman[3] points out, transformed lymphocytes or immunoblasts are characterized by basophilic nucleoli and their amphophilic cytoplasm shows strong pyroninophilia. Reed—Sternberg cells on the other hand usually exhibit strongly acidophilic nucleoli and eosinophilic cytoplasm. (This is not absolute, in that their cytoplasm can take up more of the basic stains and pyronin, in some cases.) These differences in staining characteristics are linked with cell metabolism and the majority of readily recognizable Reed—Sternberg cells are quiescent and incapable of division, contrasting with the heightened activity of transformed lymphocytes.

Histological changes similar to those following vaccination occur in herpes zoster and also in the local nodes following other immunization procedures, such as against influenza and pertussis.

Infectious Mononucleosis

This viral infection is usually accompanied by lymph node enlargement, the cervical nodes being most severely affected. Sometimes the lymphadenopathy is predominant, and therefore a node may be biopsied prior to the establishment of the diagnosis by other means. The histological appearance is variable and depends on the stage and severity of the infection. At first, the majority of the atypical lymphoid cells circulating in the peripheral blood are B lymphocytes, infected with Epstein—Barr virus nucleic acid, but after about two weeks, these lymphocytes are eliminated by the host's cellular mechanisms, and the majority of the circulating cells are then found to be T lymphocytes.

The lymph nodes show non-specific features of inflammation, with increased vascularity and swollen endothelial cells. There may be increase in size of the follicular centres, and these may be unusual in shape and contain many phagocytic macrophages[4].

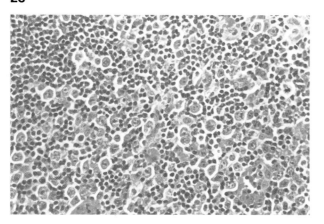

Figure 6.1 Numerous transformed lymphocytes in the paracortical area give rise to a characteristic mottled appearance. A shrinkage artefact causes the largest cells to lie within spaces. H & E ×230.

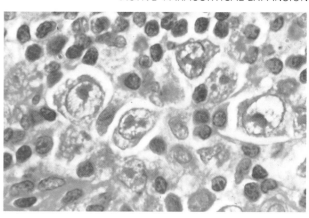

Figure 6.2 Active paracortex with transformed lymphocytes or immunoblasts. The nucleoli of these cells are fairly large and tend to be centrally placed within the nucleus. H & E ×910.

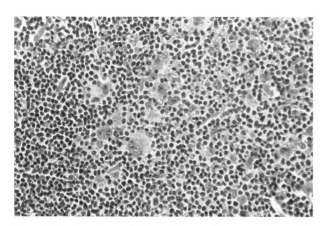

Figure 6.3 An axillary node from a 33-year-old woman with a week's history of fever, rash and lymphadenopathy. Her daughter had had a similar illness. Dilated blood vessels in the paracortex are closely related to large cells with abundant cytoplasm, polylobed nuclei and distinct basophilic nucleoli. This was interpreted as a reactive change. She remains well three years later. H & E ×230.

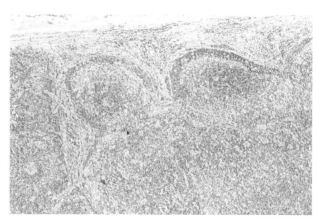

Figure 6.4. Infectious mononucleosis. Most of the changes affect the paracortical area which is relatively pale, because at this stage, numerous histiocytes are also present. Note also the considerable capsular infiltration which is present. H & E ×36.5.

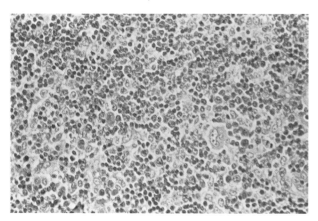

Figure 6.5 Infectious mononucleosis. Against a background of smaller lymphoid cells and histiocytes, an occasional much larger transformed lymphocyte is conspicuous. H & E ×230.

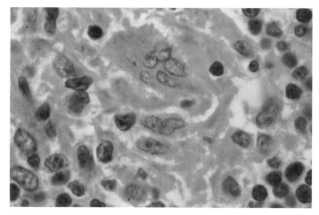

Figure 6.6 An epithelioid granuloma. H & E ×910.

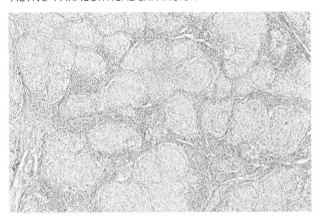

Figure 6.7 Sarcoidosis. Although granulomas may be so closely packed that lymphoid tissue is almost obliterated, they tend to remain discrete. H & E ×36.5.

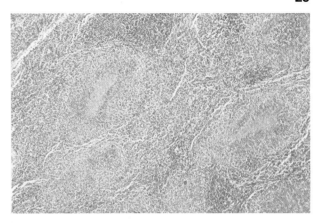

Figure 6.8 Cat scratch disease. The inguinal node from a child with a two-week history of a swelling. Conspicuous palisading of epithelioid histiocytes at the edges of necrotic areas. H & E ×36.5.

However, this is not often seen and most reports indicate a reduction in the follicles. The diffuse and often florid paracortical response, taking place at the same time, comes to overwhelm the cortical element and take over most of the node. This expanded paracortex contains lymphoid cells at all stages of development but particularly noticeable in some cases are large, atypical transformed lymphocytes. Some lie in clear spaces, with apparently little cytoplasm surrounding them and have rather open nuclei and distinct nucleoli (Figure 6.5). They can be binucleate. Others have more abundant ampho- or eosinophilic cytoplasm and huge nucleoli, described as resembling glassy inclusions, surrounded at times by perinucleolar haloes[5]. These cells of course are virtually indistinguishable from Reed–Sternberg cells.

Mitotic figures are numerous and the lymphoid cells extend through the capsule into the surrounding tissues. Small areas of necrosis occur, often having some of the more bizarre cells at their edge. Foci of histiocytes can be present and in some cases, presumably at a later stage of the disease, come to dominate the paracortical area.

The sinuses are enlarged, sometimes containing increased lymph and many lymphoid cells of primitive appearance, but in other cases, packed with a population of uniformly sized, rather featureless histiocytic cells ('immature or unripe histiocytes'), such as also occur in toxoplasmosis and brucellosis[1]. This appearance when combined with foci of histiocytes can lead to considerable overlap in the histological appearances of these conditions. In earlier stages, it may resemble the changes seen following vaccination.

However, the most important problem which arises is that of confusion with a lymphoma and these cases have not infrequently been diagnosed as such[5]. The distinction can be a difficult one. Although in infectious mononucleosis the architecture of the node can be distorted, even unrecognizable in an H & E section, a reticulin stain may show that it has not been destroyed. A more important point, however, is the extremely florid nature of the proliferation, so much mitotic activity, so much pleomorphism of the cells, vascular proliferation and endothelial cell swelling. These are all hallmarks of exaggerated reactive change; lymphomas have a less active and more monotonous appearance.

But of course the pleomorphic appearance, especially when combined with Reed–Sternberg-like cells, argues strongly for Hodgkin's disease. Although the presence of Reed–Sternberg cells is required for the diagnosis of Hodgkin's disease, in itself it is not enough. The cells have to appear in a cellular background appropriate to that condition. In infectious mononucleosis, the unusual large cells are only one end of a spectrum of appearances, most of which are consistent with transformed lymphocytes. They must be 'read in context' to understand their significance. Having this in mind, it may be possible to suspect that the condition is reactive. In any case, whether the diagnosis is confident or merely tentative, further serological investigation must be undertaken in order to confirm it.

Granulomatous Responses

Caseating Granulomas

These characterize infection with *Mycobacterium tuberculosis*, the central area of the granuloma breaking down to be replaced by eosinophilic, structureless material and surrounded by epithelioid histiocytes amongst which are the large, multinucleated Langhans giant cells. Small lymphocytes cluster around the margin of the granuloma. Coalescence of separate granulomas can take place with extensive tissue destruction.

This 'classical' picture is not always seen; at an earlier stage, there may simply be granulomas without caseation. In some patients, there is relative failure of granuloma formation, and the disease is manifested by irregular zones of necrosis, containing abundant neutrophil leukocytes, surrounded by palisaded histiocytes, and thus simulating infection by other agents (see below).

Fungal infections can give rise to a histological appearance entirely similar to that which occurs characteristically in tuberculosis. In any granulomatous condition, appropriate special stains should therefore be employed.

Granulomas with Central Necrosis

This subsection refers not to those necrotizing granulomas associated with blood vessels which reflect systemic disease, but rather to the conditions in which curiously elongated and sometimes serpiginous zones of necrosis develop, surrounded by a fringe of palisaded, epithelioid histiocytes.

One example is cat scratch disease (non-bacterial regional lymphadenitis), where the agents are still unknown and contact with cats cannot always be substantiated, but the name is familiar by usage. There are non-specific features of chronic inflammation with fibrous thickening of the capsule, through which lymphocytes extend into the surrounding tissues. Blood vessel proliferation is evident, with many migrating lymphocytes crossing their walls, and around them form clusters of histiocytes. Extremely irregular pale areas composed principally of histiocytes are randomly distributed, sometimes immediately beneath the capsule, and tend to undergo central necrosis (Figure 6.8). A few multinucleated cells of Langhans type are included in the granulomas. Sometimes transformed lymphocytes are frequent in the intervening paracortex; the follicles are inconspicuous.

In the inguinal lymph nodes, lymphogranuloma inguinale gives an entirely analogous appearance and in the mesenteric nodes, yersinial infections are similar, except that although geographical abscesses are present, there may not always be much evidence of granuloma formation.

Non-caseating, Non-necrotizing Granulomas

The best example is sarcoidosis, a disease which may be due to a transmissible agent, but none has yet been identified. The granulomas appear first in the paracortical region. They are very well defined, a feature accentuated by use of a reticulin stain, and are approximately equal in size. Even when numerous, they merely pack together, remaining as discrete entities (Figure 6.7). They rarely undergo central necrosis, but an occasional very small area may be seen.

These granulomas include multinucleated giant cells, often with Schaumann bodies. Although the latter are associated with sarcoidosis, they can be seen in other granulomatous conditions.

Foreign substances of course give rise to granulomatous responses and they include lipid, silica, beryllium, zirconium and tattoo pigment, but an important example to remember is the occurrence of granulomas in nodes draining malignant neoplasms, such as carcinomas. They can also be seen in lymphoid tissues of patients with Hodgkin's disease, even in those sites which appear to be uninvolved[6].

References

1. Symmers, W. St. C. (1978). The lymphoreticular system. In W. St. C. Symmers (ed.) *Systemic Pathology, Vol. II*, p. 563. (Churchill Livingstone).

2. Hartsock, R. J. (1968). Postvaccinial lymphadenitis. Hyperplasia of lymphoid tissue that simulates malignant lymphomas. *Cancer*, **21**, 632.

3. Dorfman, R. F. and Warnke, R. (1974). Lymphadenopathy simulating lymphomas. *Hum. Pathol.*, **5**, 519.

4. Salvador, A. H., Harrison, E. G. and Kyle, R. A. (1971). Lymphadenopathy due to infectious mononucleosis: its confusion with lymphoma. *Cancer*, **27**, 1029.

5. Tindle, B. H., Parker, J. W. and Lukes, R. J. (1972). 'Reed–Sternberg cells' in infectious mononucleosis? *Am. J. Clin. Pathol.*, **58**, 607.

6. Kadin, M. E., Donaldson, S. S. and Dorfman, R. F. (1970). Isolated granulomas in Hodgkin's disease. *N. Engl. J. Med.*, **283**, 859.

Sinus Responses and 'Passive' Paracortical Expansion

Sinus Responses

Introduction

Lymph node sinuses may be accentuated as a result of simple dilatation, or there may in addition be an increase in their cellular content. In the condition of lymphangiectasia the lymphatic vessels and sinuses are all unusually dilated but contain principally fluid, in the absence of other complications. Of course, mesenteric nodes contain a relatively dilated sinus system, since vast quantities of fluid drain from the intestine under normal circumstances.

If there is chronic venous obstruction impeding the lymphatic drainage then, besides fibrosis, the lymph node sinuses may undergo a peculiar vascularization. Haferkamp et al.[1] referred to this change as vascular transformation.

In the majority of other conditions where the sinuses appear prominent, there is an increase in their histiocyte content, which may result both from increased drainage from the periphery and proliferation within the sinuses themselves. This is referred to as sinus lining cell hyperplasia or histiocytosis and the appearance can be modified further depending upon the stimulus provoking the change.

Lastly, increase in the cell population of the sinuses may be due to their infiltration by cells other than histiocytes. Not uncommonly, these are neoplastic in nature, but may represent extramedullary haemopoiesis.

Sinus Histiocytosis

This is an extremely common change, encountered in nodes draining most inflammatory and neoplastic conditions, and often present as part of more complicated responses. Clearly this represents accentuation of one aspect of normal node function and usually lacks any specific significance. In some cases, pigmented substances may be concentrated in the sinus histiocytes such as carbon or tattoo pigment. Occasionally, sinus histiocytes are found to contain spindle shaped or ovoid brown bodies, varying from 3 μm to 10 μm in length, for the most part. They stain positively by Perls Prussian Blue method and in the PAS reaction, and probably contain both lipofuscin and iron. They have been referred to as 'Hamazaki-Wesenberg' bodies[2] and are of unknown significance, although it has been suggested that there is an association with the presence of epithelioid granulomas. Their greatest importance lies in not confusing them with other things, in particular mycotic infections.

In states of accelerated red cell breakdown, hyperplasia of sinus histiocytes occurs as part of a generalized response, and there may be evidence of erythrophagocytosis, together with haemosiderin granules within the cells. It is important to remember that this change is not uncommon, and the finding of erythrophagocytosis is not to be equated with the condition of malignant histiocytosis.

Lymphangiogram Effect

This investigation, often preceding lymph node biopsy, can produce dramatic effects, in that the lipid-based, radio-opaque material is deposited in the sinuses where it provokes a florid granulomatous response. Multinucleated giant cells of foreign body type are stretched around the rim of clear spaces from which the lipid has dissolved, and overall there is increase in the size and number of histiocytes (Figure 7.2). Usually the condition remains confined to the sinuses but may spill over into the node pulp. With the passage of time, the vacuoles disappear and the response dies down.

Lipogranulomatosis

The development of granulomas in relation to lipid materials draining to lymph nodes can occur in many situations, and the cause is easily understood. However, their development in relation to materials draining from the area of the gall bladder is less well appreciated. Usually, besides the striking bubbly appearance of the sinus histiocytes, due to their intracytoplasmic vacuoles, (Figure 7.4) bile pigment can also be seen. Clusters of histiocytes often occur outside the sinuses also and their contained lipid may escape to form extracellular globules, which in turn promote a foreign body response. Occasionally, in cases of long standing, granulomas of sarcoid type develop.

Whilst of little importance in itself, this change, because of its distribution, may be confused with Whipple's disease and the correct diagnosis should be made by recognition of the bile pigments present.

Whipple's Disease

The changes in the lymph nodes in this rare systemic disorder are not all that different from the last two described. Again, the effects are seen first in the sinuses, with increase in the size and number of histiocytes, and the development of clear cystic spaces, because lipid comes to accumulate there, and this in turn provokes a granulomatous response. The other feature however is the presence of granular material in the histiocyte cytoplasm which is strongly positive by the PAS method of staining, and which corresponds with bacillary bodies seen

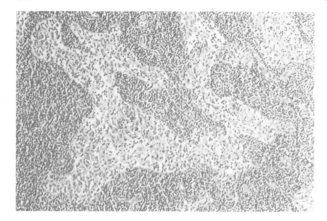

Figure 7.1 Simple sinus histiocytosis or sinus hyperplasia. H & E × 91.0.

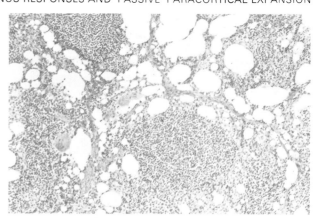

Figure 7.2 Lymphangiogram effect. A pre-operative lymphangiogram had been performed about a week before excision of this node, in which clear rounded spaces, fringed by foreign body type giant cells, distend the sinuses. H & E × 91.0.

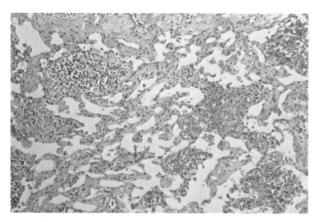

Figure 7.3 Chronic obstruction to venous drainage from a node results in gradual fibrosis of the sinuses, coupled with proliferation of the lymphatic channels, as shown here. In more extreme cases, actual vascularization of the sinuses occurs. H & E × 91.0.

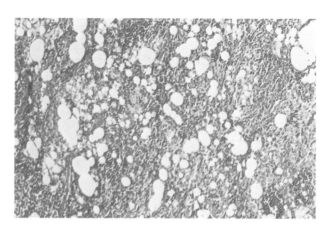

Figure 7.4 An enlarged lymph node in the upper abdomen was noted during routine palpation in the course of a cholecystectomy for gall stones. It contained abundant lipid and a small amount of yellow-brown pigment. Lipogranulomatosis. H & E × 91.0.

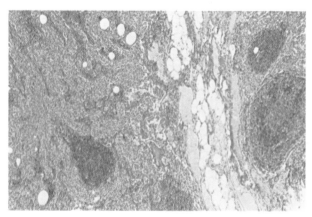

Figure 7.5 Generalized mild lymphadenopathy accompanied fever and weight loss in a 36-year-old man. There was severe depletion of normal lymphoid tissue, accompanied by densely packed histiocytes in the distended sinuses. In some areas were changes resembling immunoblastic lymphadenopathy. He was thought to have an acquired immune deficiency. H & E × 36.5.

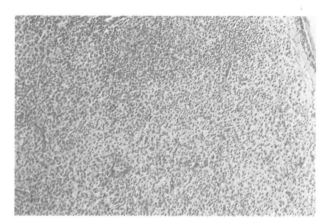

Figure 7.6 Passive paracortical expansion. The paracortical area is pale due to accumulation of bland histiocytes. H & E × 91.0.

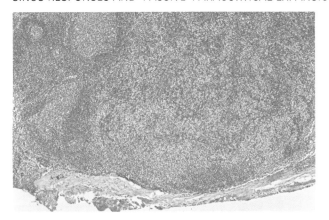

Figure 7.7 Dermatopathic lymphadenopathy. Slightly nodular expansion of the paracortical area, again with pallor attributable to histiocytes. H & E ×36.5.

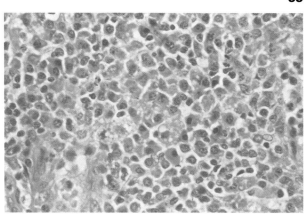

Figure 7.8 Dermatopathic lymphadenopathy. Histiocytes with lipid vacuoles and melanin granules in their cytoplasm are admixed with many plasma cells in this example. H & E ×365.

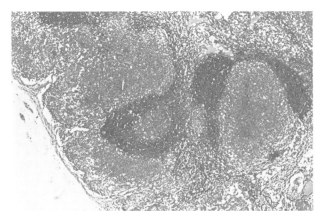

Figure 7.9 Lipidosis, Hand–Schüller–Christian disease. Histiocytes admixed with eosinophils distend the sinuses initially and later involve the node pulp. H & E ×36.5.

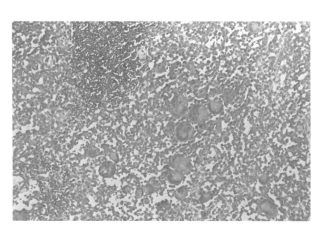

Figure 7.10 Hand–Schüller–Christian disease. Multinucleated histiocytes are commonly present, sometimes in clusters. H & E ×91.0.

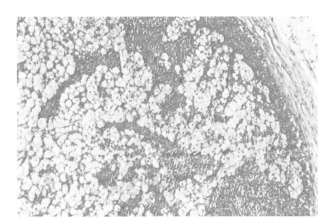

Figure 7.11 Lepromatous leprosy. Large clear histiocytes distend the paracortex. (In the early stages, Hand–Schüller–Christian disease can give a rather similar appearance). Appropriate staining in a case of leprosy shows numerous intra-cytoplasmic acid-fast bacilli. H & E ×91.0.

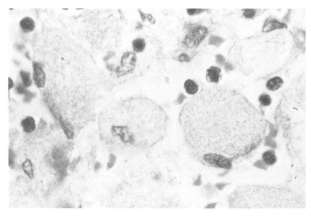

Figure 7.12 The characteristic large cells which are present in Gaucher's disease. Their cytoplasm is said to resemble crumpled tissue paper. H & E ×910.

with the electron microscope. Although the changes are most characteristic in the mesenteric nodes, the non-caseating granulomas alone are found in other nodes, such as those in the axilla[3]. The diagnosis should not be missed if the PAS stain is always done in cases of unexplained granulomatous inflammation.

Extra-medullary Haemopoiesis

In general this does not give rise to much lymph node enlargement but on the other hand is not uncommonly encountered in post-mortem lymph nodes. Recognition is usually made easy by the presence of megakaryocytes, and the eosinophil myelocytes which are usually conspicuous, even if few. The application of the appropriate esterase stain can be used to confirm the diagnosis.

Neoplastic Cells

The appearance of these varies of course with the neoplasm concerned, and their nature is usually self-evident. Whilst their proliferation may be confined within the sinuses for a while, usually there is invasion of the node itself, once the condition is established, and where there is widespread sinus involvement, the possibility of malignant histiocytosis should be considered.

'Passive' Paracortical Expansion

Introduction

This term is being used to describe conditions in which the paracortex appears greatly expanded, due to the presence of histiocytes principally. Even if the process was initiated in the sinuses, this aspect is overwhelmed by subsequent outward spread into the nodal pulp, giving a much more diffuse pattern of involvement. The word 'passive' is used to imply that the histiocytic accumulation does not appear to be primarily the result of T lymphocyte activity; it does not suggest that the histiocytic population itself is not undergoing proliferation. The population of histiocytes is capable of expansion in response to stimulation and indeed there is constant turnover of cells even in apparently 'stable' conditions. Histological appearances of this type in lymph nodes may be the result of local drainage of materials or possibly micro-organisms, usually already intracellular; or they may reflect systemic disorders where, as a result of an enzyme defect, metabolites accumulate and are stored within macrophages as well as other tissues, since there is no normal method of disposal.

Dermatopathic Lymphadenopathy

This change affects nodes draining an area of chronic skin irritation and when severe can almost obliterate the nodal architecture, which is replaced by a sheet of pale cells, leaving only follicular remnants at the edges. There is nothing in the development of this change which is specific to the skin condition itself, and it may be related to oily substances applied to the skin, together with the patient's own scratching of the area.

Often, remnants of sinus hyperplasia can be recognized, and a variable number of transformed lymphocytes may be present, since the remaining

lymphocytes are of course still capable of responses. The chief feature which enables the diagnosis to be made is recognition that some of the histiocytes contain lipid droplets and melanin granules, (Figure 7.8). This is not always easy and stains for melanin, together with a frozen section of the node stained for lipid should be undertaken in doubtful cases.

Amongst the histiocytes, there are often eosinophils, as well as neutrophils and plasma cells. This mixture of cells in the infiltrate and the presence of large transformed lymphocytes with conspicuous nucleoli, together with diffuse obliteration of architecture and failure to notice the lipid and melanin, has led to incorrect diagnosis of Hodgkin's disease in this condition. This is yet another example where the appropriate clinical history can prevent such mistakes being made, even when the histological appearance is equivocal.

A much more difficult problem arises when the clinician is uncertain as to the nature of the skin condition, previous biopsies may have failed to give a positive diagnosis, and the enlarged node is then removed to decide whether the patient has a cutaneous lymphoma. Changes of dermatopathia there may be, but if much lymphocyte transformation is also present, it can be difficult to rule out lymphoma with confidence. However, the diagnosis of mycosis fungoides should only be made when the large and bizarre nuclei characteristic of that condition have been definitely identified.

Lipidoses

Metabolic disorders due to enzyme defects result in storage of the accumulating lipid within tissues and cells, including histiocytes, and therefore the involvement of lymph nodes is only part of a generalized disease. The extent to which they may be involved is variable.

The accumulation of glucocerebrosides in Gaucher's disease leads to the appearance of large, round to oval histiocytes, which take on a more polygonal outline when pressed up against one another. Their pale cytoplasm has a characteristic appearance, said to resemble crumpled tissue paper, which is due to fine lines which appear to cross one another (Figure 7.12). Commonly some of these enlarged histiocytes are multinucleate.

In Niemann–Pick disease, sphingomyelin is stored inside cells, and again enlarged macrophages in excessive numbers characterize the disorder. The average size of the histiocytes in this condition is a little less than that of Gaucher cells, and their cytoplasm appears foamy due to the presence of fine vacuoles. Multinucleate forms are unusual.

The diagnosis of these rare disorders, with their striking clinical presentations, is unlikely in practice to rest upon a lymph node biopsy, but this may be the case in Hand–Schuller–Christian disease with unusual features and especially in eosinophilic granuloma, the solitary manifestation of the same basic disorder, which can present in lymph nodes alone[4], although this is rare.

In both conditions, although the blood cholesterol is within normal limits, cholesterol and its esters are concentrated within histiocytes, which appear somewhat enlarged, with clear pale cytoplasm. Multinucleate cells occur and may have an enormous number of nuclei. The histiocytes are found within sinuses, and as clusters in the node pulp (Figure 7.10) occasionally involving the follicles, and exhibiting a well marked granulomatous appearance at times.

The conspicuous feature however, is the admixture of eosinophil leukocytes with the histiocytes, which can be so numerous as to give rise to eosinophil 'abscesses' as described in a case of eosinophilic granuloma, by Reid et al.[4].

Lepromatous Leprosy

Almost unexpectedly, it seems appropriate to include this disease under the general heading of 'passive' paracortical expansion, and yet it equates well with the manner in which the host is overrun by these mycobacteria of low virulence, when the cellular responses are inadequate. Histiocytes appear helpless against the proliferating bacteria and are simply used to accomodate them. Thus the lymph nodes like other tissues become stuffed with enlarged histiocytes containing the bacilli (Figure 7.11). The organisms may be so numerous that they appear like bundles of twigs within the cytoplasm of the cells, easily visible even in H & E stained sections. Their acid-fast nature is demonstrable by use of the modified Ziehl–Neelsen stain.

Iatrogenic Causes of Lymph Node Enlargement

These are numerous, and although effects first appear in the sinuses, by the time enlargement is sufficient to provoke excision of the node, there is usually extensive change in the interfollicular area.

Considerable expansion due to the presence of large clear histiocytes, some of which appear to contain denser, globular material, is seen following the use of polyvinylpyrrolidone, either as the vehicle for a depot injection or intravenously. Similarly, the widely used silicone compounds lead to accumulation of large macrophages with vesicular clear cytoplasm, in some cases progressing to a granulomatous appearance.

In the absence of the relevant clinical history, interpretation of changes such as these is difficult, but unexplained histiocyte accumulations should always raise the suspicion of iatrogenic causation.

Other changes in lymph nodes, attributed to drugs, are discussed on page 38.

References

1. Haferkamp, O., Rosenau, W. and Lennert, K. (1971). Vascular transformation of lymph node sinuses due to venous obstruction. Arch. Pathol., **92**, 81.

2. Symmers, W. St. C. (1978). Lymphoreticular system. In W. St. C. Symmers (ed.). Systemic Pathology Vol. II, p. 563. (Churchill Livingstone).

3. Case Records of the Massachusetts General Hospital (Case 35, 1971). N. Engl. J. Med., **285**, 567.

4. Reid, H., Fox, H. and Whittaker, J. S. (1977). Eosinophilic granuloma of lymph nodes. Histopathology, **1**, 31.

Toxoplasmosis

Infection by *Toxoplasma gondii* is not at all uncommon and may present as lymphadenopathy[1], the cervical lymph nodes being most frequently affected. From the clinical point of view, it is often felt that the patient has a lymphoma and particular responsibility rests with the surgical pathologist in this instance to recognize the nature of the condition. Otherwise the patient will receive inappropriate therapy with possibly tragic results.

If it is felt that there is even a possibility that the condition could be due to toxoplasmosis, this should be stated, since the diagnosis can be confirmed by serological testing. The causative organisms are present within the lymphoid tissue, but have only rarely been demonstrated[2,3].

Follicular hyperplasia occurs, but not all the follicles need be affected. Generally, they are increased in number and in particular they are large and bizarre in outline, often dumb-bell shaped, with considerable evidence of nuclear breakdown, and phagocytosis of the debris by macrophages. This gives a striking low-power 'starry' appearance, but, in addition, there are loose clusters of epithelioid histiocytes scattered through the interfollicular areas, sometimes more numerous towards the periphery of the node. These extend into the follicular centres themselves and this feature is extremely suggestive of toxoplasmosis, although it does also occur in leishmaniasis (Figure 8.6).

A third component of the histological picture is the distension and packing of sinuses in the outer part of the node (including the marginal sinus), with fairly large cells resembling monocytes (occasionally admixed with some lymphocytes and neutrophils). Lennert has referred to this by the evocative term 'unripe sinus histiocytosis' (Figure 8.2). Other accompanying changes are thickening of the capsule and increase in the size of endothelial cells in both capillaries and venules.

Conditions in which somewhat similar histological appearances can occur are brucellosis, early cat scratch disease and even infectious mononucleosis. At times too, there can be a very real confusion with histiocyte predominant Hodgkin's disease, because later in the course of toxoplasmosis the appearance of the node comes to be dominated by the clusters of histiocytes throughout it. At the same time, there may still be scattered, large transformed lymphocytes, together with plasma cells in the medulla, and acceptance of the reactive lymphoid cells as Hodgkin's cells leads to the erroneous diagnosis.

Leishmaniasis

Occasionally this disease presents as enlargement of lymph nodes, without other features. The histological appearances are very similar to those of toxoplasmosis, in that clusters of histiocytes, often epithelioid in type, are distributed through the nodes and may extend into the follicular centres. However, they often include multinucleate giant cells and closely resemble non-caseating tuberculoid granulomas. Careful examination however, reveals the presence of Leishman–Donovan bodies within the cytoplasm of the macrophages (visible in an H & E stained section) although on histological grounds alone these cannot be distinguished from other similar parasites[4].

Plasma cells with Russell bodies may be numerous in the interfollicular areas and medulla and also infiltrate the capsule, together with lymphocytes and occasional multinucleate giant cells.

Syphilis

The enlarged lymph nodes in this infection show a combination of host responses to spirochaetes, which disseminate via the blood-stream. Sections stained by the Warthin–Starry method demonstrate the organisms lodged in blood vessel walls or within the follicular centres themselves[5]. On the whole, the cervical, occipital and axillary nodes show only follicular hyperplasia, although the reactive centres are often very large and lack the usual rounded configuration. Phagocytic macrophages often give a conspicuous 'starry-sky' appearance. These changes may be confused with follicular lymphoma[6].

The most severe changes occur in the inguinal nodes; in addition to follicular hyperplasia, there is thickening and fibrosis of the capsule which is infiltrated by plasma cells, especially in perivascular distribution. Plasma cells form a conspicuous feature in the rest of the node as well, but in addition there may be a florid arteritis (Figure 8.10) with neutrophil leukocyte infiltration or the classical change of endarteritis obliterans. The paracortex may appear pale because of relative decrease in lymphocytes and infiltration with histiocytes. In a number of cases definite granulomas of tuberculoid type occur, and these seem to be related to the presence of persistent spirochaetes. The possible relationship of this persistence, and relative lymphocyte depletion, is discussed by Turner and Wright[7].

Systemic Lupus Erythematosus

Rarely, this condition presents as lymph node enlargement, which may be considerable and involves the cervical nodes to the greatest extent. Where the diagnosis is entirely unsuspected clinically, it poses a very real problem, since pathognomonic histological features are not always present.

Firstly, there is follicular hyperplasia, the follicular edges sometimes looking a little blurred. Phagocytic macrophages impart a starry-sky pattern to the follicles. The interfollicular area presents an untidy appearance and is much expanded. It contains small blood vessels proliferating amongst lymphocytes and numerous plasma cells, between which eosinophilic collagen may be closely interweaved. In places it has a spotty appearance due to pale histiocytes and some of these are multinucleate, with up to 5 or 6 nuclei (Figure 8.8).

There may be considerable fibrosis. One case showed marked thickening of the capsule, which was infiltrated by plasma cells, together with dense fibrotic bands within the pulp of the node, apparently related to blood vessels. This gave a 'nodular sclerosing' appearance. Concentric rings of fibrosis surround small arteries, again with plasma cells interleaved (Figure 8.7), and in some areas increasing fibrosis, laid down in a random fashion, gradually overtakes the node.

Plasma cells remain entrapped within it. Here and there are eosinophilic Russell bodies; eosinophils are virtually absent. The sinuses may simply be filled with small lymphocytes but sometimes the sinus histiocytes are large and multinucleate and can show considerable erythrophagocytosis.

In more florid cases, there are areas of necrosis. Haematoxyphil bodies, composed of broken down nuclear material and antibody, may be seen. There may even be virtual replacement by necrotic debris and haematoxyphil bodies, but this extreme change is rare in biopsy material.

Only the presence of haematoxyphil bodies can be said to be definitely indicative of systemic lupus erythematosus, in a lymph node biopsy, since they are probably related to the LE cell phenomenon. Occasionally, indeed, one may see these homogenized, rounded bodies pushing the nucleus of a phagocytic cell to one side, exactly as may be demonstrable in the incubated blood of these patients[8]. In the absence of these findings, it may be very difficult to reach any definite diagnostic conclusion. The peculiar perivascular sclerosis may lead one to think in terms of a 'connective tissue disease', but failing this, the important point is to recognize that although there is overall blurring of architectural features by the cellular infiltrate and the fibrosis, there is no true destruction of the node, except in the rare cases showing extensive necrosis. Moreover, the presence of so many mature plasma cells points to a reactive process.

Lymphadenopathy Attributed to Drugs

This has been reported most frequently in association with treatment by hydantoin derivatives in cases of epilepsy, but other drugs have occasionally been implicated and these include penicillin, sulphonamides and some anti-inflammatory agents such as phenylbutazone. The reaction usually occurs within seven to ten days after commencing drug therapy, but some reports have suggested that it can be delayed for more than a year.

Lymph node changes are only a part of what appears to be a generalized hypersensitivity response and the patients also have fever, skin rashes, and hepatosplenomegaly, together with anaemia, leukopaenia and an increase in plasma cells in the bone marrow and peripheral blood. In most cases lymph node enlargement is widespread, with the cervical nodes being most affected, but a case having a single, enlarged node in the neck has been reported. The increase in size of the nodes can take place rapidly and the cut surfaces may show macroscopic areas of haemorrhage and necrosis.

The severity of histological changes engendered is variable. The follicles and their centres persist, but do not appear to contribute any particular proliferative activity. A somewhat pleomorphic cellular and vascular reaction replaces the normal nodal tissue, giving rise to differing degrees of effacement of the architecture[9]. Thus blood vessels appear numerous and prominent with many large transformed lymphocytes having pyroninophilic cytoplasm, some of which are definitely plasmacytoid in appearance, and in addition there are mature plasma cells, eosinophils, histiocytes and neutrophils in varying proportions. Some of the large lymphoid cells are atypical and may even be multinucleate. Lastly, small foci of necrosis can occur and even frank infarcts, associated with arteritis and thrombosis.

Histologically at least there are some features in common with immunoblastic lymphadenopathy (pages 47–50) but, in contrast, the often acute, drug-induced changes almost always regress when the drug is withdrawn. The extremely pleomorphic appearance blurring the normal features, together with large atypical cells of multinucleated type, may easily be confused with lymphoma, particularly Hodgkin's disease. The knowledge that the patient is taking anticonvulsants is paramount in reaching the correct diagnosis and if no history of drug therapy has been given, then the pathologist who encounters this histological appearance must enquire carefully for himself.

Lymphomas of both Hodgkin's and non-Hodgkin's types have occurred in patients on anticonvulsant therapy[10, 11], but this was mostly of several years' duration[11]. However, it is important to remember that if nodal enlargement persists after withdrawal of the drug, a further biopsy should be carried out to exclude the possibility that the patient has indeed developed a lymphoma.

Whether drugs capable of giving rise to these hypersensitivity responses are really also responsible for neoplastic development remains uncertain[12]. The histories of the patients described by Hyman and Sommers[11] did not suggest a preceding period of lymphadenopathy. Indeed, looking at the parallels, insofar as they may be drawn, with immunoblastic lymphadenopathy, it would seem most likely that the lymphomas induced would be immunoblastic sarcomas. The possible carcinogenic role of the anticonvulsant drugs is discussed by Kruger and Harris[13] on the basis of their results using mice as an experimental model. In strains both with a tendency to spontaneous lymphoreticular neoplasia and without, they found an increased tendency to the development of lymphomas, and felt that there was both overstimulation and atrophy of immunocompetent tissues, as a result of phenytoin administration. It is not yet known whether similar effects occur in man.

Vasculitis

Disorders affecting principally blood vessels can be

39

reflected in lymph nodes, which may be biopsied if they become enlarged. This is particularly likely to occur if the vasculitis is accompanied by granuloma formation. The majority of these disorders are the direct result of immune responses, although the detailed mechanisms are not yet clear. Injuries may be due to direct attack on the components of vessel walls, or complexes can be deposited within the walls with consequent complement damage, or the reaction may take place outside the vessel wall itself. In the main, it is arteries of differing size which exhibit the lesions, and there is often an overall distribution characteristic of each disease syndrome. However, in what has been referred to as hypersensitivity angiitis there may also be involvement of the veins and, in one such case, the presentation was that of a single enlarged lymph node, showing almost exclusively venous lesions (Figure 8.11).

The affected vessels show either fibrinoid necrosis or cellular infiltration of their wall, often not involving the entire circumference. Fibrin is deposited in the extravascular tissues (Figure 8.11) and extensive granulomas, often infiltrated by eosinophils, are formed. These granulomas may invade the follicular centres and resemblance to the response in toxoplasmosis is furthered by the finding of an increase in the so-called 'immature histiocytes' in marginal sinuses. Such observations are all pointers to the fact that the patterns of granulomatous response, by which specific infections are recognized, simply form part of basic immunological responses to certain antigens. Patients in whom there are changes of this type may have a previous history of allergic diseases, or have been exposed recently to drugs[14].

11. Hyman, G. A. and Sommers, S. C. (1966). The development of Hodgkin's disease and lymphoma during anti-convulsant therapy. *Blood,* **28**, 416.
12. Editorial (1971). Is phenytoin carcinogenic? *Lancet,* **2**, 1071.
13. Kruger, G. R. F. and Harris, D. (1972). (Letter). *Lancet,* **1**, 323.
14. Rosenberg, T. F., Medsger, T. A., DeCicco, F. A. and Fireman, P. (1975). Allergic granulomatous angiitis (Churg–Strauss syndrome). *J. Allergy Clin. Immunol.,* **55**, 56.

The figures relating to this chapter are on pages 40 and 41.

References

1. Dorfman, R. F. and Remington, J. S. (1973). Value of lymph node biopsy in the diagnosis of acute acquired toxoplasmosis. *N. Eng. J. Med.,* **289**, 878.
2. Stansfeld, A. G. (1961). The histological diagnosis of toxoplasmic lymphadenitis. *J. Clin. Pathol.,* **14**, 565.
3. Stanton, M. F. and Pinkerton, H. (1953). Benign acquired toxoplasmosis with subsequent pregnancy. *Am. J. Clin. Pathol.,* **23**, 1199.
4. Daneshbod, K. (1978). Localised lymphadenitis due to Leishmania simulating toxoplasmosis. Value of electron microscopy for differentiation. *Am. J. Clin. Pathol.,* **69**, 462.
5. Hartsock, R. J., Halling, L. W. and King, F. M. (1970). Luetic lymphadenitis: a clinical and histological study of 20 cases. *Am. J. Clin. Pathol.,* **53**, 304.
6. Evans, N. (1944). Lymphadenitis of secondary syphilis. Its resemblance to giant follicular lymphadenopathy. *Arch. Pathol.,* **37**, 175.
7. Turner, D. R. and Wright, D. J. M. (1973). Lymphadenopathy in early syphilis. *J. Pathol.,* **110**, 305.
8. Moore, R. D., Weisberger, A. S. and Bowerfind, E. S. Jr. (1957). An evaluation of lymphadenopathy in systemic disease. *Arch. Int. Med.* **99**, 751.
9. Saltzstein, S. L. and Ackerman, L. V. (1959). Lymphadenopathy induced by anticonvulsant drugs and mimicking clinically and pathologically, malignant lymphomas. *Cancer,* **12**, 164.
10. Gams, R. A., Neal, J. A. and Conrad, F. G. (1968). Hydantoin-induced pseudo-pseudolymphoma. *Ann. Int. Med.,* **69**, 557.

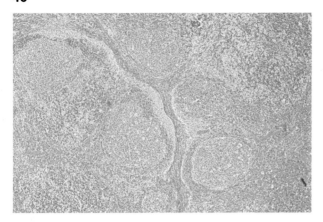

Figure 8.1 Toxoplasmosis. Expansion of the paracortex with pale histiocytes, follicular hyperplasia and cells distending the sinuses are all appreciable on low power examination. H & E   ×36.5.

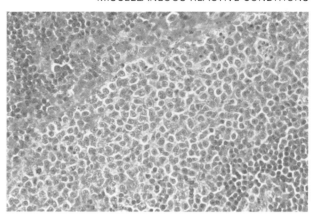

Figure 8.2 Toxoplasmosis. The sinuses are filled by closely packed, slightly angulated cells. So-called immature or 'unripe' sinus histiocytosis. H & E   ×230.

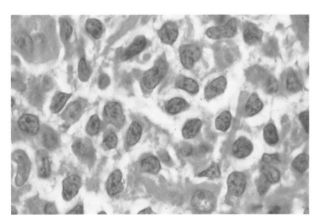

Figure 8.3   'Unripe' sinus histiocytosis in toxoplasmosis. H & E   × 910.

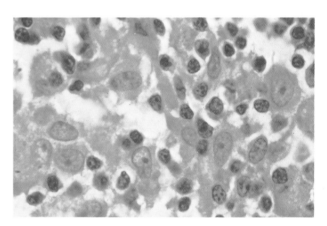

Figure 8.4   The common form of sinus histiocytosis, to compare with Figure 8.3. H & E   ×910.

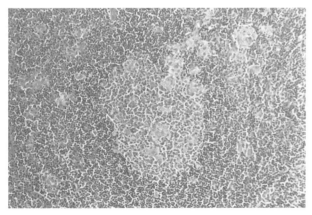

Figure 8.5   Toxoplasmosis. Clusters of histiocytes in the paracortical area and also extending into a follicular centre. H & E   ×36.5.

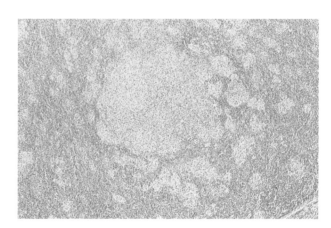

Figure 8.6   Leishmaniasis. An appearance exactly similar to that in toxoplasmosis. Figure 8.5. H & E   ×36.5.

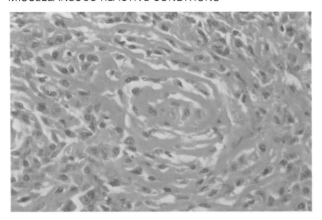

Figure 8.7 Systemic lupus erythematosus. Blood vessels surrounded by concentric laminae of collagen with interleaved plasma cells. H & E ×365.

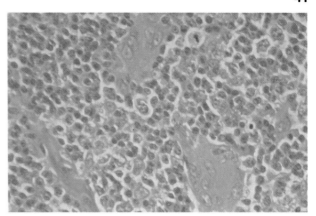

Figure 8.8 Systemic lupus erythematosus. In other areas, sheets of plasma cells with some plasmablasts and multinucleate histiocytes. H & E ×365.

Figure 8.9 Epanutin effect. In this case, the changes are indistinguishable from other examples of active paracortical response. Immunoblasts give a 'starry-sky' appearance and there is blood vessel proliferation. H & E ×91.

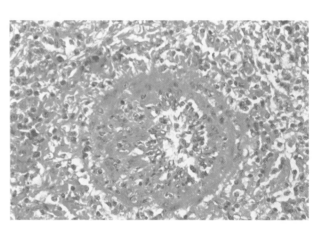

Figure 8.10 Syphilis. An inguinal node removed from a young man contained densely packed plasma cells surrounding small blood vessels. Arterioles are almost blocked by endothelial cell swelling and proliferation, with associated vasculitis. H & E ×230.

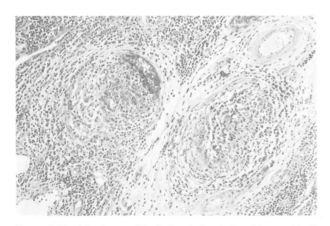

Figure 8.11 Allergic vasculitis. An inguinal node in a 14-year-old girl became enlarged and painful. There were severe vascular lesions restricted almost entirely to veins, with eccentric deposits of fibrin adjacent to the lumen, accompanied by dense cellular infiltration. H & E ×91.

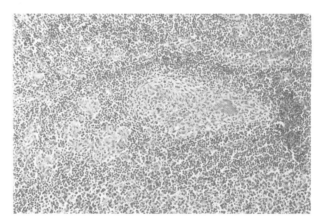

Figure 8.12 Allergic vasculitis. In the same node as that shown in Figure 8.11, there were granulomas. These extended occasionally into follicular centres. H & E ×91.

Reactive Changes Versus Neoplasia

The interpretation of the changes which occur in lymph nodes can be extremely difficult. The difficulties however are perhaps not so great as dogma inherited from the past suggests, since that dogma was based upon the fact that lymph node function was incompletely understood. However, still there occurs a steady trickle of really intriguing cases which defy a wholly confident assessment.

The first requirements, before any opinion can be expressed, are purely technical. As already stressed, adequate fixation, without prior distortion of the tissue due to manipulation, and excellent histological preparation are essential. Whilst really clear-cut conditions can be diagnosed even through the fog of less-than-perfect material, others cannot, and to give a definite opinion based on inadequate evidence is dangerous.

The other absolute requirement, in any particular case, is to obtain the relevant clinical history. Florid and puzzling changes can result from the effects of drugs and artificial immunization for example, and it is foolish not to garner every possible scrap of helpful information before arriving at a firm diagnosis.

Adequate sampling of the tissue must be carried out; if not required for other purposes, the entire node or nodes may be blocked and sectioned. The importance of using a preparation to show reticulin, in assessment, has been stressed already. (Perhaps not as useful as a radiograph for examining a chest but it should be thought of in those terms!)

The foregoing considerations apply to any case in point; then there are those which relate to the observer, who must approach the problem with a clear concept of both reactive changes and features of neoplasia, so that he has a background against which to judge the unknown. Also included in this background must be an awareness of those abnormal responses, the histological appearances of which are now recognized, although the mechanisms are not yet clearly understood.

Often the decision as to whether a given node shows a reactive or a neoplastic change rests upon a careful evaluation of the low-power appearance. Increase in size of a node is almost always due to an increase in the cell population and the first objective is to assess whether this increase is associated with any of the functional compartments. There may be a very obvious follicular component and, especially in the early stages, recognition of neoplastic follicles may be difficult (Figure 9.1). Reactive centres are usually extremely clear-cut in appearance against the surrounding corona of lymphocytes. They do not always have a rounded outline and at high power appear pleomorphic.

Follicular lymphomas tend to be more monoto-nous both cytologically and in overall appearance, most of the structures having a round or oval shape. Sometimes a lymphocyte corona is present (Figure 9.1) but more often it is not. An artefactual splitting of the section around the circumference of the neoplastic follicles, related to differing density of the tissues is often a helpful feature, and the reticulin shows compression of the pre-existing framework by the newly grown nodules (Figure 9.3). Maintenance of the follicular pattern in spread of the neoplasm outside the capsule is especially useful (Figure 9.5).

Alternatively, the increased population in the node may confine itself to sinuses and/or paracortex. If histiocytes are numerous, is there some straightforward explanation for their presence in the shape of lipid vacuoles or pigment granules?

Is the basic architecture intact, distorted or destroyed? Degrees of distortion can occur in exaggerated reactive responses and even blurring of normal zones of activity, as in infectious mononucleosis (Figure 9.8). On the other hand, the architecture can be perfectly preserved, and yet the normal elements have melted away before a diffuse infiltration of cells, such as occurs in less aggressive and usually small-celled neoplastic processes such as chronic lymphocytic leukaemia and cases of Waldenström's macroglobulinaemia.

An essential criterion for recognizing neoplastic change is the relative monotony of the cell population (Figure 9.6). Neoplastic cells result from the uncontrolled proliferation of a malignant clone and are closely related to one another, whereas reactive states represent complex co-operative activity between differing cell types, and thus result in a more mixed appearance.

The above statements preclude of course Hodgkin's disease, which is anything but monotonous, exhibiting not only variety in the form of its neoplastic cells, but also in the extravagant cellular reactions which occur about them. However, in the other forms of lymphoma the concept of monotony is a useful one. It can even be applied to those proliferations characterized by large and small nuclei (mixed lymphoma) or containing bizarre and very large nuclei. The lower power impression is still one of uniformity in a sheet of cells, lacking functional organization.

Spread of cells beyond the capsule of the node can be helpful. Admittedly, lymphoid cells stray into the adjacent adipose tissues in many reactive conditions, but this is an irregular process and there may be definitive clusters present, or a perivascular distribution. In neoplastic states, often a diffuse sheet of cells spreads out uniformly and, as it were, mindlessly, through the surrounding tissues. The

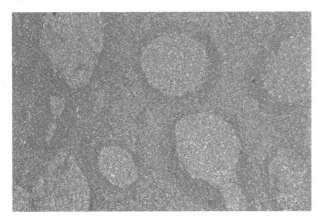

Figure 9.1 The enlarged cervical and axillary nodes from a 25-year-old man contained numerous follicular structures differing little from normal follicular hyperplasia, except that they were uniformly distributed throughout the node and large cleaved cells seemed unusually numerous. Later biopsies were of unequivocal follicular lymphoma. H & E ×36.5.

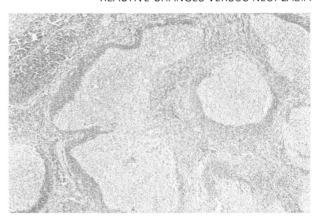

Figure 9.2 Just as bizarre forms of follicular hyperplasia occur (Figure 5.5), equally they may be encountered in follicular centre cell lymphomas. This example also has partial lymphocyte mantles present. H & E ×36.5.

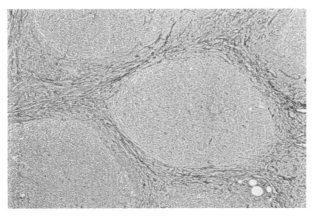

Figure 9.3 Follicular lymphoma. A section stained to demonstrate reticulin fibres may show compression of the pre-existing nodal tissue by expanding neoplastic nodules. Reticulin ×36.5.

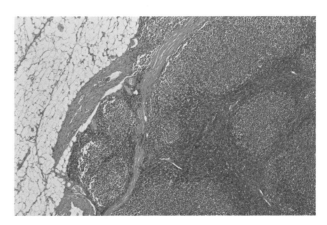

Figure 9.4 Follicular lymphoma. In this example there is beginning to be loss of follicular pattern and bands of sclerosis are developing. Another helpful diagnostic feature is the maintenance of nodularity as adipose tissue is invaded. H & E ×36.5.

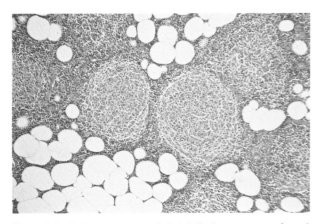

Figure 9.5 Follicular lymphoma. Orderly follicular structures are formed, but there is a tendency to cytological monotony and obvious invasion of adipose tissue. H & E ×91.

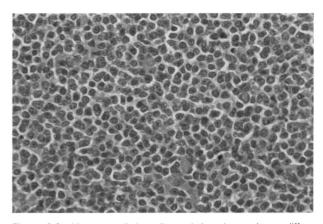

Figure 9.6 Monotony of the cell population characterizes a diffuse lymphoma composed of small, slightly irregular lymphoid cells, resembling cleaved follicular centre cells (see page 71). H & E ×365.

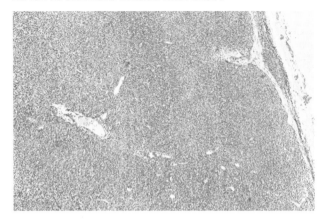

Figure 9.7 Obliteration of normal components by a diffuse small cell lymphoma. At one edge there is capsular infiltration. H & E ×36.5.

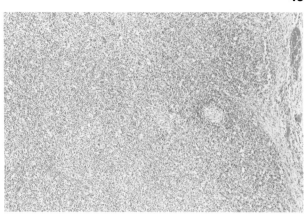

Figure 9.8 Similar virtual effacement of pattern can occur however in reactive conditions, as shown here in a case of infectious mononucleosis. This is accompanied by cellular infiltration of the capsule, but it is scanty and ragged compared with that seen in Figure 9.7. H & E ×36.5.

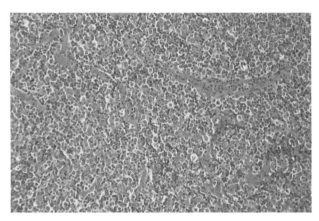

Figure 9.9 An enlarged mesenteric lymph node was removed from a child, at the time of appendicectomy. The blood vessels are conspicuous with egress of numerous lymphocytes and the histological appearance is dominated by large lymphoid cells. This active paracortical response could be confused with a lymphoblastic lymphoma. H & E ×91.

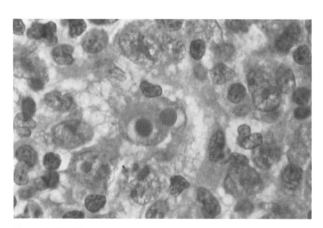

Figure 9.10 The same node shown in Figure 9.9 contained a few cells of this appearance, with hard edged large nucleoli surrounded by clear haloes. Cells indistinguishable from Reed–Sternberg cells are reported in infectious mononucleosis but the Paul–Bunnell reaction was negative in this case. H & E ×910.

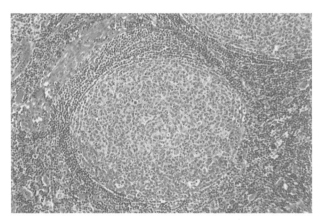

Figure 9.11 (This and Figure 9.12 are from the same case). A 45-year-old man had his enlarged cevical lymph nodes removed. There were numerous large follicular structures dispersed throughout, but the majority of them could not be differentiated from reactive follicular centres, as illustrated here. H & E ×91.0.

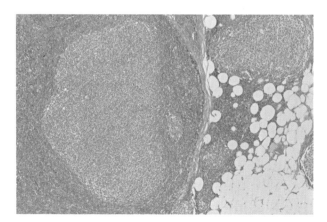

Figure 9.12 One or two of the follicular structures were however larger and had a more monotonous cellular composition. In addition, examination of further blocks of tissue showed nodular extension into adipose tissue in the centre of the node. No treatment was instigated in this case and four years later, the patient remains symptom free. H & E ×36.5.

increased ease of recognition of follicular lymphoma has already been mentioned.

Where the nodal architecture has been destroyed, it is usually easy to recognize whether or not this is due to a neoplastic process, since the reactive changes causing such damage are usually unmistakable, with areas of necrosis and fibrosis.

Having decided that the process is neoplastic, the question of excluding non-lymphomatous tumours arises. Where there is only partial involvement of the node, there is no difficulty, in that the distinction between a metastatic deposit and normal lymphoid tissue is usually clear-cut, and this may be accentuated by compression of adjacent tissue, contrasting with the intimate mixture of normal components with their own lymphomatous variants. But diffuse nodal replacement by a poorly differentiated non-lymphomatous tumour can be much more difficult to recognize. The decision must rest upon whether the cells appear to be cohesive, whether they form nests or acinar structures and on their cytological features, together with any evidence of function, such as mucin secretion or presence of melanin granules.

Where it is concluded that the neoplasm is a lymphoma, besides the easily recognized follicular pattern evidence of others must be sought, such as a pseudofollicular arrangement due to proliferative centres, or coarsely nodular modes of growth, as occur in Hodgkin's disease. The low-power examination also gives an excellent idea of the size range of the dominant cells in the proliferation. By the time the observer proceeds to the detailed cytological assessment (and this should include using the oil immersion objective), most of the fundamental decisions should have been made, and the details of the cells will come to be those expected, rather than a revelation, particularly with experience.

Lastly, there are those nodes which show neither normal response patterns nor frank neoplasia, and yet their appearance is abnormal. Perhaps this is best explained as a lack of organization, in that there is unusual blood vessel proliferation, accompanied by what are normal cell constituents, but these are in disorderly arrangement. Features such as these characterize abnormal immune reactions. Apparently normal events at the cellular level are incoordinated overall and this accords well with concepts of these diseases, which imply defects in the normal control of immunological responses.

Introduction

Quite apart from the normal reactive responses and frankly neoplastic conditions, there are disorders associated with abnormality in immunological function. They are important from the clinical aspect, and because they predispose to the development of neoplasia; but in the present context their importance lies in their unusual histological appearances, probably often misinterpreted in the past.

Considered under this heading are immune disturbances, both congenital and acquired. The first group consists of rare disorders, usually clearly recognized on clinical grounds and presenting in early life, but the second group has been less well understood and only recently became better defined. Although patients with acquired hypogammaglobulinaemia had been well appreciated, it was not until a few years ago that a disease of another group of patients, middle-aged or elderly for the most part, was recognized[1, 2]. These patients fail to produce orderly, and therefore effective, responses to antigenic stimulation, which results clinically in undue susceptibility to infection, and evidence of unwanted end-products, in the shape of high levels of serum immunoglobulins. The term immunoblastic or angioimmunoblastic lymphadenopathy has been applied to disorders of this type.

The status of angiofollicular hyperplasia, or giant lymph node hyperplasia, remains an enigma but it is included in this section, since in some cases there are systemic symptoms similar to patients with immunoblastic lymphadenopathy. Also, in that it represents a disordered arrangement of lymphoid tissues, there are also histological parallels.

Congenital Immune Deficiencies

Although these conditions are usually recognized clinically, a lymph node biopsy may be carried out as part of the detailed investigation, since precise diagnosis is required for genetic counselling, as well as for treatment. Examination of an unstimulated node may give little information and the procedure is of most value if preceded by prior stimulation. The findings correspond with what is known of lymph node function. Thus in B lymphocyte defects with lack of immunoglobulin, follicular centres and plasma cells are absent; in thymic deficiency, no paracortical response can be elicited, and in those rare cases of severe combined immunodeficiency, the excised tissue proves to be merely a fibrotic anlage, with some histiocytes and a few lymphocytes within it. Lymphocyte depletion, increasing in severity with age is found in the cortex and paracortex in the immunodeficiency syndrome associated with ataxia–telangiectasia, and in the paracortical areas of nodes from patients with the Wiskott–Aldrich syndrome. In the latter condition

there is failure to respond to certain polysaccharide antigens.

In some patients, the block in B lymphocyte development occurs at a later stage. Webster[3] refers to a case of primary hypogammaglobulinaemia in which there was actually increase in the number of germinal centres, but complete absence of plasma cells.

Acquired Immunological Defects

(1) Unlike the congenital form, **hypogammaglobulinaemia** is not sex-linked in distribution and occurs later in life. The clinical history is often one of recurrent episodes of infection. Again the histological appearance reflects interference with normal B cell development. Some cases exhibit follicular centres only, with complete absence of plasma cells, and it is important to differentiate this pattern from follicular lymphoma[4], but in the majority the follicles undergo atrophy[5].

Interestingly enough, these patients often have epithelioid granulomata with multinucleated giant cells, which may be seen in the lymph nodes as well as the liver and spleen. It has been postulated that this response is the one which develops in the absence of the normal activity of immunoglobulin[6].

(2) **Immunoblastic (angioimmunoblastic) lymphadenopathy** patients exhibit disorganized immunological responses, reflected both in the histological appearance of lymphoid tissue and in the clinical features. Besides lymphadenopathy, which is usually generalized, they have hepatosplenomegaly, fever, skin rashes, polyclonal hypergammaglobulinaemia and often haemolytic anaemia. A certain number of patients give a history of recent exposure to drugs which perhaps precipitate the condition.

Both the histological and clinical features suggest that there is excessive proliferation of B lymphocytes. Whether this is due to a relative failure to monitor the 'switching-on' of B lymphocytes, or an inability to terminate their activity is not clear. One explanation of the abnormality is that the defect is actually within the T cell population, and this is the most widely held view at the present time.

The prognosis for the majority of patients with this condition is grave. Many succumb to infections and a high proportion of them, not surprisingly, in view of the florid proliferation which occurs, evolve to lymphoma[7] (Figure 10.12). This is either of immunoblastic type or composed of cells showing definite plasmacytoid change. It has been difficult to establish the ideal form of treatment in these cases; this may well be due to the facts that this is probably not an entirely homogeneous group and that the development of lymphoma may not always be demonstrable in the tissues examined.

The alternative name used to describe the con-

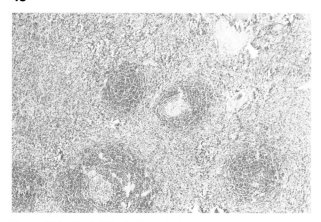

Figure 10.1 Angiofollicular hyperplasia of hyaline vascular type. The entire tissue consists of structures resembling normal follicles. Collagenous thickening surrounds larger blood vessels in the intervening areas. H & E ×36.5.

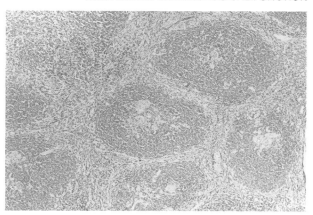

Figure 10.2 Angiofollicular hyperplasia. This example conforms more to the plasma cell type, in that many of the paler areas in the centres of the follicles, at higher power, show considerable resemblance to follicular centres. H & E ×36.5.

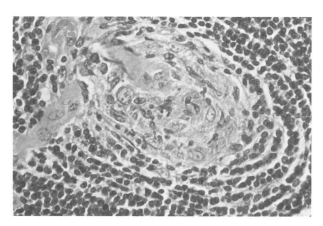

Figure 10.3 Angiofollicular hyperplasia, hyaline vascular type. A hyaline thick walled blood vessel is surrounded by fairly large pale cells, against which serried ranks of lymphocytes are arranged. The appearance suggests some bar to the normal development of a follicular centre. H & E ×365.

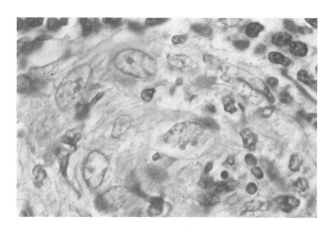

Figure 10.4 Angiofollicular hyperplasia, hyaline vascular type. The cells which surround the central hyaline blood vessel resemble dendritic reticular cells. H & E ×910.

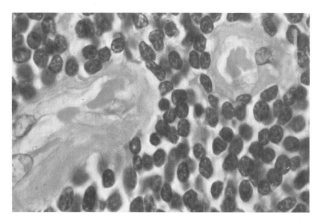

Figure 10.5 Angiofollicular hyperplasia, hyaline vascular type. In the 'inter-follicular' areas, small blood vessels, with thick hyaline walls are surrounded by small lymphocytes. H & E ×910.

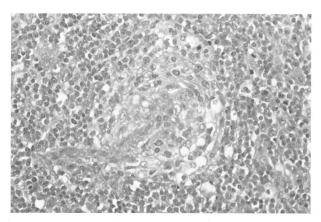

Figure 10.6 Immunoblastic lymphadenopathy. A pseudo-follicular structure, one of several present in this case, bears a close resemblance to those in angiofollicular hyperplasia. H & E ×230.

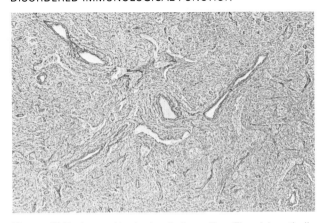

Figure 10.7 Immunoblastic lymphadenopathy. The rich reticulin network, often showing a concentric arrangement around the vascular elements, differs from the pattern in a normal node. Reticulin ×91.0.

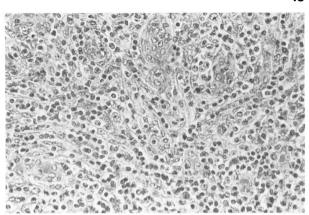

Figure 10.8 Immunoblastic lymphadenopathy. This shows the swirling pattern of blood vessels, formed of plump endothelial cells, lying amongst lymphoid cells of variable size and appearance. H & E ×230.

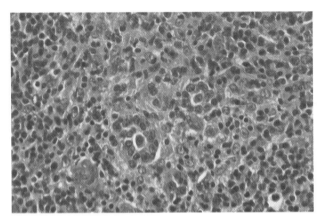

Figure 10.9 Immunoblastic lymphadenopathy. In this example, from one of the enlarged nodes in a 56-year-old man, this rather unusual phenomenon was noted. Rings of intermediate sized lymphoid cells are arranged around central larger cells, which also appear to be lymphoid in nature. H & E ×230.

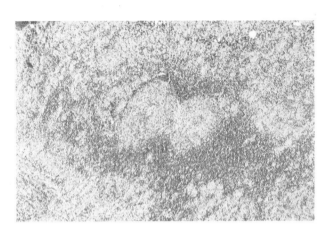

Figure 10.10 (Figures 10.10 to 10.12 are all from the same patient). A mass in the axillary tail of a middle-aged woman consisted of small lymphocytes, and histiocytes in clusters. It was interpreted as lymphocyte predominant Hodgkin's disease on the basis of larger lymphoid cells present. On review at this centre, a perivascular distribution of histiocytes was noted. H & E ×36.5.

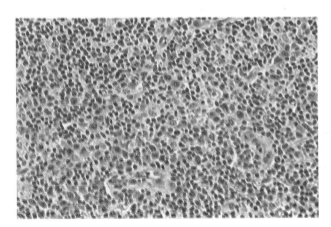

Figure 10.11 A cervical node removed at the same time was interpreted as immunoblastic lymphadenopathy when reviewed and it was felt that the axillary lesion must be considered as another part of the same disorder. H & E ×230.

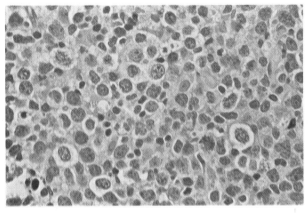

Figure 10.12 The cervical node also included, however, areas such as this, where the appearance was dominated by large cells, often in mitosis and it was felt that this was early evidence of evolution to immunoblastic lymphoma. H & E ×365.

dition, angioimmunoblastic lymphadenopathy, emphasizes the proliferating blood vessels which characterize the histological appearance. Vascular proliferation is seen in reactive changes but, in these nodes, normal structures are replaced by leashes of blood vessels, often in a swirling pattern, which are shown up well either in a reticulin stain (Figure 10.7) of a PAS preparation. The latter is positive because vessel walls are often thickened by basement membrane-like material deposited within and around them[8]. Amongst the vessels are many resembling post-capillary venules, by virtue of their tall endothelial cells (Figure 10.8).

Clustered around the blood vessels, sometimes in linear arrangement, are lymphoid cells showing all stages of the later development of B lymphocytes, from immunoblasts to mature plasma cells. The precise composition of this cell population varies from case to case; one included tubular array plasma cells[9], but cytologically they resemble cells found in reactive nodes[8]. Eosinophils, sometimes numerous, are present in the infiltrate and histiocytes too occur as a variable component, often of epithelioid type, and may be arranged in clusters.

Another feature of varying prominence, is intercellular, amorphous, PAS positive material, much of which consists of cytoplasmic fragments[10], although other material is also present. In two cases recently reported[10], amyloid was demonstrated both within such deposits and around blood vessels, but this is unusual. A decision as to whether or not what may be an extremely florid proliferation, including numerous immunoblasts, has become neoplastic in nature, is not always an easy one. Nathwani et al.[7] used the criterion of finding clusters of large lymphoid cells within blood vessels as an early indication of lymphoma.

The peculiar and conspicuous vascular proliferation which occurs in this condition provokes considerable speculation. Similar vessels, with tall endothelial cells, are seen in graft rejection (and an early impression of the entire disorder was that it resembled a graft-versus-host reaction[1]); it has been suggested that they develop as a result of activity by lymphoid cells, either directly or indirectly[11].

The pleomorphic histological appearance in this condition has been confused with Hodgkin's disease, particularly because amongst the immunoblasts there may be much larger cells, with correspondingly large or multiple nuclei (see Chapter 11).

Other histological features occur and no doubt increasing sophistication in methods of investigation will reveal qualitative differences in the defects which occur. About a third of the cases reported by Frizzera et al.[1] had 'burnt-out' follicular centres in the cortex and they described and illustrated aggregates of dendritic reticular cells, either well-vascularized or appearing rather like epithelioid granulomas. Cases such as these appear to provide evidence of a close relationship with the entity of angiofollicular hyperplasia, discussed below.

Angiofollicular Hyperplasia (Giant Lymph Node Hyperplasia)

This unusual condition, which can generate tumours of considerable size, has been described most frequently within the thoracic cavity, but other sites, including extranodal ones, may be affected. In a recently reported case, the lesions were multicentric and included splenic involvement[12].

There are two histological sub-types recognized and the first, the so-called plasma cell type, found in only about 10–20% of the total reported cases, is associated with a clinical syndrome of fever, hypergammaglobulinaemia and anaemia. Alleviation of this syndrome usually follows excision of the mass which often includes a rim of compressed normal node. The rest of the tissue consists of follicular centres, occasionally containing acidophilic material, separated by densely packed plasma cells and immunoblasts permeated by tortuous blood vessels.

Possibly this active appearance evolves to the hyaline–vascular type seen in the majority of cases. In these, the follicular structures have a central, thick-walled vessel associated with large cells and surrounding concentric layers of lymphocytes (Figure 10.3). The intervening tissue contains numerous small blood vessels which are often hyaline and there may be considerable deposition of collagen around larger blood vessels as well as areas of fibrosis. Lymphocytes predominate in the population but plasma cells, immunoblasts and eosinophils also occur.

Many of the cases reported have been single localized tumours, and it has been suggested that they simply represent lymphoid hamartomata. However, the occurrence of systemic symptoms, other similarities to immunoblastic lymphodenopathy, the fact that structures resembling these 'pseudofollicles' may sometimes be seen in reactive nodes, and the recently reported multicentric case, all argue that these tumours result from localized, abnormal responses to certain stimuli. The pattern of distribution suggests that these stimuli are encountered most frequently via the lungs, but probably the intestinal tract is similarly involved.

References

1. Frizzera, G., Moran, E. M. and Rappaport, H. (1974). Angioimmunoblastic lymphadenopathy. *Lancet*, **1**, 1070.

2. Lukes, R. J. and Tindle, B. H. (1975). Immunoblastic lymphadenopathy. A hyperimmune entity resembling Hodgkin's disease. *N. Engl. J. Med.*, **292**, 1.

3. Webster, A. D. B. (1977). Immunodeficiency. In E. J. Holborow and W. G. Reeves (eds.). *Immunology in Medicine: A comprehensive Guide to Clinical Immunology*, pp. 473–535. (New York: Grune & Stratton, London: Academic Press).

4. Lukes, R. J. and Collins, R. D. (1974). Immunologic characterisation of human malignant lymphomas. *Cancer*, **34**, 1488.

5. Rosen, F. S. and Janeway, C. A. (1966). The gamma globulins. III. *N. Engl. J. Med.*, **275**, 709.

6. Prasad, A. S., Reiner, E. and Watson, C. J. (1957). Syndrome of hypogammaglobulinaemia, splenomegaly and hypersplenism. *Blood*, **12**, 926.

7. Nathwani, B. N., Rappaport, H., Moran, E. M., Pangalis, G. A. and Kim, H. (1978). Malignant lymphoma arising in angioimmunoblastic lymphadenopathy. *Cancer*, **41**, 578.

8. Neiman, R. S., Dervan, P., Haudenschild, C. and Jaffe, R. (1978). Angioimmunoblastic lymphadenopathy. An ultrastructural and immunologic study with review. *Cancer*, **41**, 507.

9. Averback, P. (1977). A human tubular array plasma cell. *Virchows Arch. A. Path. Anat. Histol.*, **377**, 17.

10. Madri, J. A. and Franowitz, F. (1978). Amyloid deposition in immunoblastic lymphadenopathy. *Hum. Pathol.*, **9**, 157.

11. Graham, R. C. (1974). Pathogenesis of vascular proliferation in angio-immunoblastic lymphadenopathy. *Lancet*, **2**, 666.

12. Gaba, A. R., Stein, R. S., Sweet, D. L. and Variakojis, D. (1978). Multicentric giant lymph node hyperplasia. *Am. J. Clin. Pathol.*, **69**, 86.

11

Hodgkin's Disease (Hodgkin's Lymphoma)

Introduction

Previous controversy as to the nature of this condition is still reflected in its name, but nowadays, it is widely accepted as a neoplastic disorder. However, the underlying nature of the peculiar, proliferating cells, the classical Reed–Sternberg cells and their variants, remains uncertain.

It can be argued strongly that they are lymphoid in origin, in that extremely similar large cells, apparently immunoblasts, are seen in virus infections. It is also claimed that ultrastructurally there are close resemblances to immunoblasts[1], although elsewhere more of a likeness to histiocytes is asserted[2].

The initial recognition of immunoglobulin within the cytoplasm of Reed–Sternberg cells (See Figure 2.8) suggested at first that they must be derived from B lymphocytes, but the presence of both types of light chain within a single cell make this unlikely. There is much recent evidence to suggest that the neoplastic cells of Hodgkin's disease derive in fact from histiocytic precursors; such evidence derives from studies of the cells in culture[3,4]. The use of a metalophil method by Curran and Jones[5] indicates that many of the Reed–Sternberg cells are possessed of delicate dendritic processes. This latter observation leads them to suggest that the neoplastic precursors may be the normal dendritic reticular cells of the lymph node. The presence of intra-cytoplasmic immunoglobulin would then be explained by internalization of such material, which had become attached to the surface of the cells. This could either represent a remnant of normal dendritic reticular cell function, or alternatively it is possible that tumour-specific antibody is produced by the host, and that the neoplastic cells are capable of taking it into their cytoplasm.

The undoubted fascination of Hodgkin's disease, for clinicians and pathologists alike, lies in the many guises which it can adopt. Although this variation could prove to be linked to whatever may be the initiating stimulus, it seems reasonable at present to assume that it represents differences in host response.

Excellent and detailed accounts of the histological features and current methods of classification have been given elsewhere: the classification put forward by Lukes and Butler[6] in 1966, its modifications for clinical application[7], and an extremely lucid re-appraisal by Lukes[8] in 1971.

The term, Reed–Sternberg cells (R–S cells), which is applied to the neoplastic component of Hodgkin's disease, refers to the two observers who described them at the turn of the century. 'Classical' and variant forms are both recognized. These differing forms, together with the variable host responses, in terms of cells and their products, which surround them, form the basis for the histological classification of the condition. Even before the modern classification was introduced, the relationship of histological appearance and the clinical aspects was well appreciated.

This account deals only with the aspects of Hodgkin's disease as it affects lymph nodes, and for detailed descriptions the reader is recommended to the papers of Lukes and Butler[6] and Lukes[8].

Cell Types

Reed–Sternberg cells can be viewed as the 'thumb-print' of the disease, but without a background appropriate to Hodgkin's disease they are not sufficient to make the diagnosis. Entirely similar cells have been observed in infectious mono-nucleosis[9] and other neoplastic conditions[10] and they occur in other apparent viral infections, having negative Paul–Bunnell reactions.

Classical or diagnostic R–S cells are large and their nuclei are either divided into lobes or they are multinucleated. Bi-nucleate or 'mirror-image' forms occur (Figure 11.1). The nucleoli are usually described as 'huge', with a rather homogeneous appearance, staining reddish-purple in an H & E preparation and often looking hard-edged against a clear perinucleolar halo. The nuclear membrane is thick and threads of chromatin sometimes radiate outwards from the nucleolus towards it. The cytoplasm is abundant and its staining characteristics vary from being acidophilic to amphophilic. There can be intense pyroninophilia of both cytoplasm and nucleolus. These diagnostic R–S cells are end-stage cells, incapable of further division and apparently having a derangement of their RNA metabolism. They probably give rise to the dying or mummified cells which often accompany them (Figure 11.1). Lukes[8] stresses that it is the frequency of these diagnostic Reed–Sternberg cells which provides the important prognostic factor in cases of Hodgkin's disease, rather than the proportion of lymphocytes, although these are usually inversely related.

A mononuclear variant of the diagnostic cell is probably the chief proliferative element; extremely similar cells are encountered quite commonly, however, in reactive conditions and these therefore cannot be relied upon for diagnostic purposes.

In the nodular sclerosing variety of Hodgkin's disease, lacunar R–S cells occur, named because of the artefact which develops when the tissues are fixed in formal–saline. They are large cells with abundant, often pale, watery-looking cytoplasm,

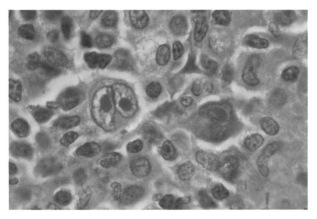

Figure 11.1 A binucleate, classical Reed–Sternberg cell, together with a similar cell undergoing degeneration. Note the reddish-purple staining of the nucleoli. H & E ×910.

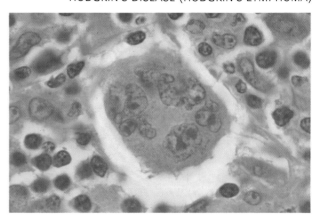

Figure 11.2 A large cell with a polylobed nucleus, lying within an artefactual 'lacuna'. Nucleoli are easily distinguished but are irregular and lack sharp margins. Cells of this type are characteristic of nodular sclerosing Hodgkin's disease. H & E ×910.

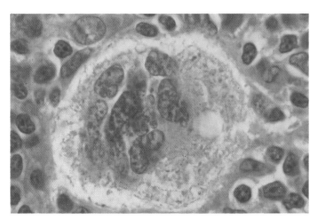

Figure 11.3 Another large cell in nodular sclerosing Hodgkin's disease but lacking a surrounding 'lacuna'. The abundant cytoplasm is rather granular and includes a rounded clear area, resembling a lipid vacuole. H & E ×910.

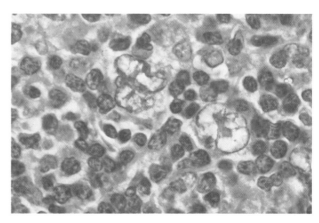

Figure 11.4 Lymphocyte predominant Hodgkin's disease with occasional abnormal cells whose delicate vesicular nuclei include distinct, but not particularly enlarged nucleoli. H & E ×910.

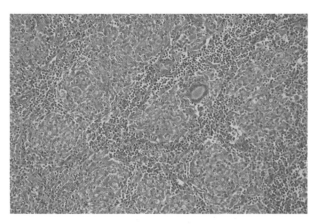

Figure 11.5 Lymphocyte predominant Hodgkin's disease, accompanied by florid granulomatous response. The diagnosis of lymphoma was overlooked in the initial biopsy on this case. H & E ×91.0.

Figure 11.6 Lymphocyte and/or histiocyte predominant Hodgkin's disease. The underlying nodularity is readily appreciable in this field. H & E ×36.5.

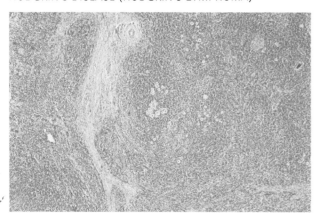

Figure 11.7 Nodular sclerosing Hodgkin's disease. The lacunar cells in this example are conspicuous. This node also includes a well developed fibrous band containing a blood-vessel. H & E × 36.5.

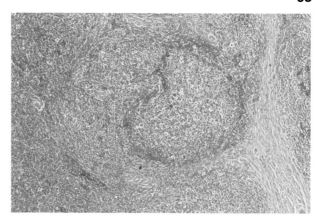

Figure 11.8 Nodular sclerosing Hodgkin's disease. The nodular character is accentuated by the development of surrounding collagenous bands. H & E × 36.5.

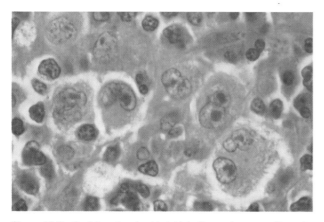

Figure 11.9 Nodular sclerosing Hodgkin's disease. Lacunar cells can be numerous and close packed, giving rise to what has been referred to as a 'cellular' variant. H & E × 910.

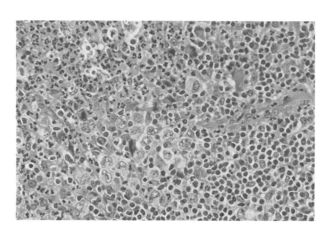

Figure 11.10 Not infrequently such 'cellular' nodules undergo necrosis and plasma cells may be numerous in the encroaching infiltrate. H & E × 230.

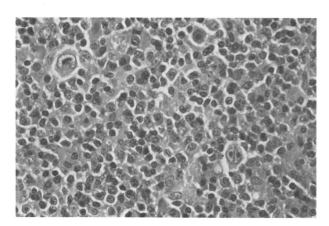

Figure 11.11 Hodgkin's disease, mixed cellularity. Bi- and mononuclear Reed–Sternberg cells are found readily and the infiltrate includes plasma cells and eosinophils. H & E × 365.

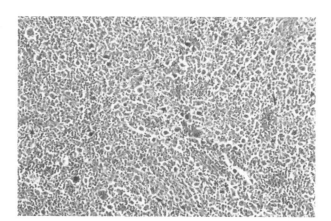

Figure 11.12 A case of Hodgkin's disease, mixed cellularity, in which conspicuous increase in the number of Reed–Sternberg cells indicates progression towards lymphocyte depletion. H & E × 91.

although sometimes it can be granular (Figure 11.3) and during formalin fixation, either it shrinks, or lipid dissolves out, leaving a clear space around the cell, the lacuna' (Figure 11.2). The nuclei of these cells are often extremely hyperlobated and their nucleoli are extremely distinct, often brightly acidophilic, but not particularly large.

In the less aggressive forms of Hodgkin's disease, lymphocyte and/or histiocyte predominant, another variant of the R–S cell occurs. This has been referred to as polyploid in type. These are fairly large cells with a nucleus of complex and folded, or somewhat twisted appearance. The nucleoli are distinct, but quite small and the chromatin is delicate and lacy. Cytoplasm is moderate in amount and rather pale. It is often difficult to recognize these cells, which can be 'tucked away' in the closely investing infiltrate (Figure 11.4), and careful examination of a thin section is required.

Lastly, in the sarcomatous variant of lymphocyte depleted Hodgkin's disease, the R–S cells can take on an extremely bizarre and pleomorphic appearance, but they usually still exhibit the same large and sharply defined nucleoli as the diagnostic cells.

Classification

On clinical and histological grounds, the nodular sclerosing category is separated from all the other cases which then, in essence, exhibit a spectrum of appearances and behaviour, from a favourable end, where R–S cells are few and lymphocytes and/or histiocytes predominate in the host's responses, to more aggressive forms of the disease in which R–S cells are usually numerous, and lymphocytes diminish There is little doubt that some individual patients can move through the spectrum, whilst others already have aggressive disease at the time of presentation.

At the Rye Conference[7], it was decided to refer to the favourable forms of the disease as lymphocyte predominant, the aggressive disease as lymphocyte depleted, and cases in between as 'mixed cellularity'. The original classification however contained six categories as explained below.

Lymphocyte Predominance

Both lymphocytes and histiocytes contribute to the background appearance and either cell type can predominate, but lymphocytes do so more commonly. This whole group was originally separated into two categories, one diffuse in nature but the other exhibiting nodularity, which is accentuated by use of a reticulin stain. The latter pattern is seen usually where lymphocytes predominate, is more likely to be associated with localized disease and thus has better prognosis.

As already stated, the polyploid type of R–S cell is associated with this sub-type and can be frequent, forming up to 10% of the population. Their recognition should promote a diligent search for diagnostic R–S cells and this may require the examination of several thin sections before one can be identified. If, on the other hand, diagnostic R–S cells are found readily, despite abundant lymphocytes in the background, the case should be classified as mixed cellularity; this is the class towards which the histological appearance is changing, and accords better with the subsequent behaviour.

Generally, very few eosinophils are present and there is no necrosis or fibrosis.

Mixed Cellularity

This type lacks definite positive attributes and to some extent functions as the category in which to place cases not reaching the criteria laid down for the other types. Diagnostic Reed–Sternberg cells are readily identified and the background infiltrate is composed of a whole mixture of cell types in differing proportions. These include lymphocytes, histiocytes, eosinophils and plasma cells. In addition there are foci of necrosis and there can also be patches of fibrosis.

Lymphocyte Depletion

This combines two of the original sub-types under one heading. Firstly, the condition of diffuse fibrosis in which cellular depletion of the lymph nodes is related to severe immunological failure clinically. The appearance is not that of 'fibrosis' in the usually accepted sense, but rather amorphous eosinophilic material is deposited in the node, and gradually takes on a more hyaline appearance. A reticulin stain shows that fibres are laid down in haphazard distribution. R–S cells may be scarce, often distorted between the eosinophilic material and recognition of diagnostic cells can be difficult. Occasional areas though can resemble the other original sub-type which is included under this same heading, the reticular type. This can be pictured evolving from the mixed cellularity type, with great increase in the R–S cells (Figure 11.12), so that they come to dominate the picture and, as they do so, the host cellular infiltrate falls away. In some cases, the R–S cells become extremely bizarre and the appearance is then that of a pleomorphic sarcoma in which it may be quite difficult to find diagnostic cells.

Nodular Sclerosing Hodgkin's Disease

This sub-type is histologically distinct from the other three, and this appears to have clinical parallels. Two of its distinctive features are referred to in its name; the atypical cells are found as aggregates and increasing fibrotic thickening of the surrounding node capsule is accompanied by extension from it of collagenous septa which extend into the node and separate the aggregates from one another. This results in the formation of nodules, separated from one another by broad bands of dense fibrous tissue, wrapped around them in a concentric fashion.

The other diagnostic feature is the presence of lacunar cells, within the nodules. In what appears to be the early stage, lacunar cells alone may be seen in the node pulp, before any fibrous bands have appeared. Probably it is unwise to make a definitive diagnosis of nodular sclerosing Hodgkin's disease on the basis of lacunar cells alone, unless it has already been demonstrated at another site in the same patient, although one may suspect that the nodular sclerosing form will evolve. In practice, firm diagnosis should rest on at least one well developed band of fibrosis (Figure 11.7).

In some centres, it is this sub-type which is encountered most frequently, but it is a far from homogeneous entity. There is enormous variation in the cell populations to be found within the actual nodules, and in essence they parallel to some extent the changes described in the sub-types outside the nodular sclerosing category. Particularly striking are those cases where the abnormal cells are numerous and appear close-packed, with relative diminution in lymphocytes; this has been referred to as the 'cellular' type (Figure 11.9). It is not uncommon for these 'cellular' nodules to undergo necrosis (Figure 11.10) and subsequent fibrosis can replace the entire nodule. It is important to recognize that these are lacunar cells. Failure to do so can result in a mistaken diagnosis of lymphocyte depleted Hodgkin's disease, with its very different prognostic implication. In cases of difficulty, connective tissue stains will accentuate the essentially nodular nature of the disease and sclerotic bands.

This category remains separated clinically and histologically from the rest, and the nodular sclerosing pattern is maintained in sequential biopsies. As already stated, there is considerable variation in the cellular composition from case to case and, at present, the most accurate prognostic implications appear to be linked to the relative proportions of lymphocytes present. It may also be that an individual patient evolves through changes similar to those that occur in the non-nodular sclerosing categories, although it is difficult to document this in practice.

Granulomas in Hodgkin's Disease

The development of granulomas in association with Hodgkin's disease is well recognized[11]. Quite separate from the granulomatous response to material injected during the course of a lymphangiogram, these granulomas can be found not only in affected nodes but also in remote tissues without apparent involvement. This has been noted particularly since the introduction of the staging laparotomy procedure[12]. They have been observed most frequently in cases of nodular sclerosing Hodgkin's disease but occur also in lymphocyte predominance. Indeed, their overwhelming presence in this form of the disease can lead to mistakes in diagnosis, the lymphoma being entirely overlooked (Figure 11.5).

At the present time, the granulomas seem to be only one more facet of the host responses, engendered by the presence of the neoplastically transformed cells of Hodgkin's disease. Prognostically, their presence does not seem to have any significance.

Nodularity in Hodgkin's Disease

Besides the extremely obvious focal pattern of growth which characterizes the nodular sclerosing variant, a variable nodular pattern can be noted in other forms of the disease, particularly in the lymphocyte predominant category. It is of some interest therefore that Curran and Jones[5] have suggested that the neoplasm is one of dendritic reticular cells. In normal lymphoid tissue, these function as the component which organizes follicular aggregation, and indeed are present within follicular lymphomas. It seems entirely feasible that they should be closely related, at least in some way, to the same phenomenon in Hodgkin's disease.

Prognosis in Hodgkin's Disease

Prognosis depends both upon the histological sub-type and the extent of disease at the time of presen-tation. These are however found to be interrelated, in that the most favourable histological sub-types are associated with least extensive tissue involvement.

The lymphocyte predominant appearance, particularly of nodular configuration, appears to represent early and restrained disease and correspondingly has the best overall prognosis. Nodular sclerosing patterns are the next most favourable, although variation is encountered in this group, and this may eventually be linked more certainly with variations in the histological appearance.

Where the responses are those of mixed cellularity and lymphocyte depletion, these seem to represent progressing disease on the one hand, and overwhelming disease on the other, and accordingly the prognostic implications are unfavourable.

Problems in the Diagnosis of Hodgkin's Disease

In considering this aspect, it is necessary to reflect upon the nature of Hodgkin's disease itself. To some extent, its separation from the other lymphomas is somewhat artificial; its positive diagnosis being a somewhat stereotyped reaction to the presence of certain abnormal cells combined with patterns of host response. But an underlying true understanding of the disease is still lacking, and only when this has been achieved will it be possible to relate Hodgkin's disease to the rest of the lymphomas, and also to assess some of the less clear-cut histological appearances which are encountered.

Commencing with the more straightforward issues, firstly there is the possibility of failing to make the diagnosis. This is most likely to occur whilst the disease is only mildly aggressive, so that failure to recognize the large, rather delicate Reed–Sternberg variants, may lead to an impression of lymphocytic lymphoma. Alternatively, the neoplastic nature may be entirely overlooked, since histiocytes and possibly granulomas dominate the picture.

Next, as has been referred to frequently in different sections of this book, there is a tendency to over-diagnose Hodgkin's disease. There are numerous conditions in which large cells of differing origins occur in lymph nodes, as often as not in combination with some eosinophils or histiocytes. Many of these, where the rigid criteria adopted in defining Reed–Sternberg cells are not adhered to, have been designated 'some form of Hodgkin's disease'. At the present time, this is to be deplored since the aggressive therapy appropriate to Hodgkin's disease is of course dangerous in itself, and may be particularly so in some disorders mistaken for Hodgkin's disease.

Probably it is forms of angioimmunoblastic lymphadenopathy which have been most often confused; indeed the extremely pronounced reactive picture, in parts of a node not yet involved by Hodgkin's disease, may be very reminiscent of this type of lymphadenopathy, with proliferating blood vessels and abundant plasma cells. In relation to the neoplastic areas themselves, plasma cells may be seen compressed between laminae of collagen, and the arteries show perivascular concentric rings of collagen, reminiscent of the 'onion-skin' appearance shown in other disorders.

Occasionally cases present themselves where, even with concepts of angioimmunoblastic lymphadenopathy and Hodgkin's disease both clearly in

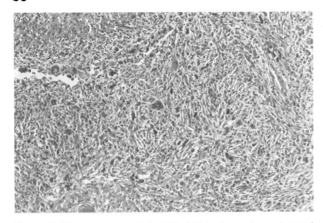

Figure 11.13   Lymphocyte depleted Hodgkin's disease. Large abnormal cells, some of which show nuclear features of Reed—Sternberg cells are present within fibrous tissue which still contains lymphocytes, but these are few in number. H & E   × 91.

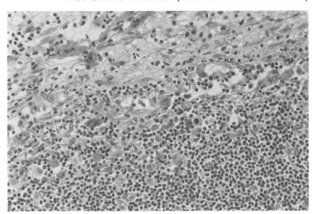

Figure 11.14   Nodular sclerosing Hodgkin's disease. Earliest involvement of a node adjacent to one in which the fully established disease was present. Reed—Sternberg cells are seen within afferent lymphatic vessels, the subcapsular sinus and invading the node pulp. H & E   × 91.

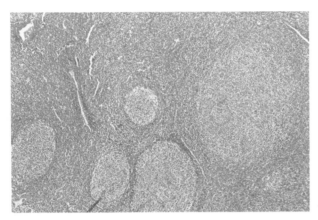

Figure 11.15   (Figures 11.15 to 11.17 are from the same patient). In one area of this node there are well defined follicular structures together with a larger blurred nodule. The appearance suggests a follicular centre cell lymphoma. H & E   × 36.5.

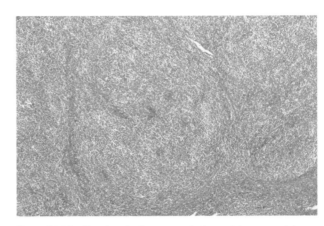

Figure 11.16   Elsewhere in the same node the nodules are much looser textured and are composed of mainly lymphocytes with some histiocytes and occasional larger cells. The appearance is very reminiscent of lymphocyte predominant Hodgkin's disease. H & E   × 36.5.

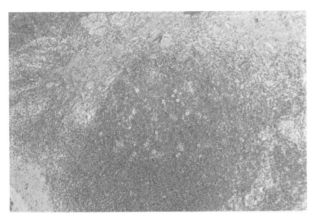

Figure 11.17   Again in the same node are areas which tend to be divided up by bands of fibrosis and scattered large cells are surrounded by lacunae. This appearance, too, is much more that of a pattern associated with Hodgkin's disease. H & E   × 36.5.

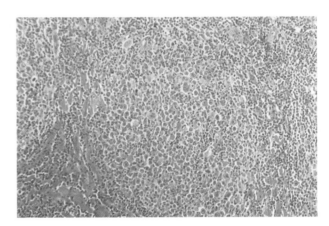

Figure 11.18   This axillary node from a 44-year-old man was classified as a follicular lymphoma. However the cells contributing to the nodular areas, have abundant eosinophilic cytoplasm, nuclei which are often polylobed and contain distinct nucleoli. They resemble closely the cell types in 'cellular' forms of nodular sclerosing Hodgkin's disease. H & E   × 91.

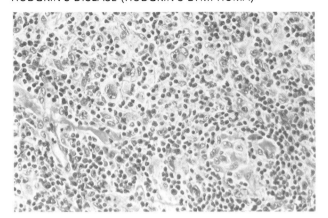

Figure 11.19 (Figures 11.19 to 11.21 are from the same case). A man of 53 years complained of fever and weight loss. A polyclonal increase in γ-globulins was demonstrated. Following a diagnosis of probable Hodgkin's disease on a cervical node, laparotomy was performed. A para-aortic node, illustrated here, showed proliferating blood vessels, intercellular deposits of PAS-positive material and a range of lymphoid cells. These are features suggestive of immunoblastic lymphadenopathy. H & E　×230.

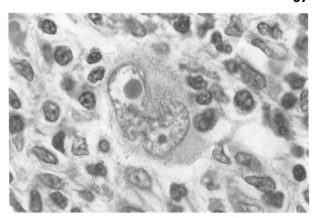

Figure 11.20 Some of the larger cells in the para-aortic node however resemble Reed–Sternberg cells. H & E　×910.

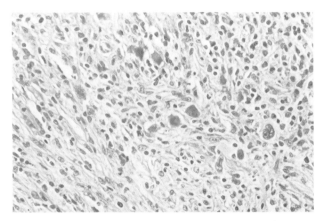

Figure 11.21 The enlarged spleen contained white nodules, some more than 1 cm diameter. Histologically these had the appearance of lymphocyte depleted Hodgkin's disease and the patient has been treated as having this condition. H & E　×230.

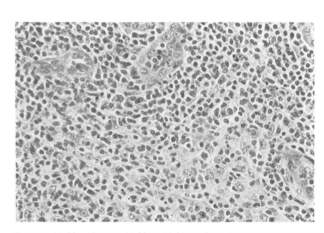

Figures 11.22 (Figures 11.22 to 11.24 are from the same patient and again illustrate parallels between immunoblastic lymphadenopathy and Hodgkin's disease). A man of 57 years was diagnosed as having nodular sclerosing Hodgkin's disease in a cervical node and a staging laparotomy was performed in this centre. The para-aortic nodes showed an appearance compatible with immunoblastic lymphadenopathy, illustrated here. H & E　×230.

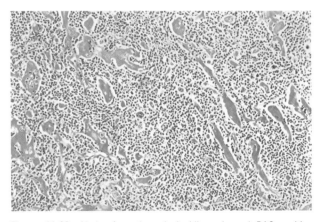

Figure 11.23 Nodes from the splenic hilum showed PAS positive material within thickened blood vessel walls and present as deposits. The background consists of small lymphocytes with scattered large cells containing polylobed nuclei. H & E　×91.

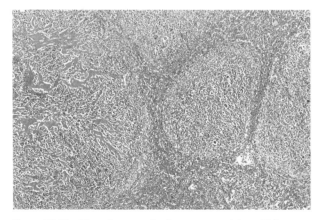

Figure 11.24 The spleen contained numerous nodules, which superficially resemble nodular sclerosing Hodgkin's disease. However atypical features are large amounts of eosinophilic and PAS positive homogeneous material deposited within the nodules and at high power, the large cells lack the cytological features of lacunar cells. H & E　×36.5.

confident conclusion (Figures 11.19 to 11.24). The suspicion arises that recognition of what is called Hodgkin's disease is based on a normal host response, and that if this is lacking, then the full-blown, 'classical' picture does not evolve.

Two types of appearance can give rise to this particular diagnostic problem, distinguishing between Hodgkin's disease and a disordered immunological response. In one there is a swirling pattern of fibrous tissue, in which blood vessels are not unduly conspicuous, but numerous large, bizarre and distorted nuclei are present. This is strongly suggestive of lymphocyte depleted Hodgkin's disease, but the pattern is inappropriate. Secondly, where the process has a vaguely nodular character, with some larger, abnormal cells towards the central part of the nodule. These may be few, and frequently their nuclei are distorted or appear to be undergoing degeneration, showing the features seen in 'mummified' Reed–Sternberg cells, but no diagnostic R–S cells are present. Sometimes, there are more large cells however, and the impression is one of failure to form a normal follicular centre.

Lastly, another group of cases, which is in some ways similar. In these, although there may be areas of undoubted follicular centre cell lymphoma, some of the follicles are much larger and blurred in appearance, (Figures 11.15 to 11.17). Their background population is one of small lymphocytes, with a few eosinophils and histiocytes, against which larger cells are conspicuous and occasionally lie in 'lacunae'. The low power diagnosis of such areas appears quite straightforward, considered in isolation. However, these large cells do not have features of classical Reed–Sternberg cells.

Therefore nodular patterns of abnormal cellular proliferation, strongly reminiscent of Hodgkin's disease, but having apparent relationships with both follicular lymphoma and immunoblastic lymphadenopathy are encountered from time to time. Although not easy to understand at the present time such cases, by their very existence, may eventually contribute to achieving a better overall understanding of lymphomas in general.

References

1. Glick, A. D., Leech, J. H., Flexner, J. M. and Collins, R. D. (1976). Ultrastructural study of Reed–Sternberg cells. *Am. J. Pathol.*, **85**, 195.

2. Lutzner, M. A., Hobbs, J. W. and Horvath, P. (1971). Ultrastructure of abnormal cells in Sezary syndrome, mycosis fungoides, and parapsoriasis en plaque. *Arch. Derm.*, **103**, 375.

3. Kaplan, H. S. and Gartner, S. (1977). 'Sternberg–Reed' giant cells of Hodgkin's disease: cultivation in vitro, heterotransplantation and characterisation as neoplastic macrophages. *Int. J. Cancer*, **19**, 511.

4. Long, J. C., Zamecnik, P. C., Aisenberg, A. C. and Atkins, L. (1977). Tissue culture studies in Hodgkin's disease. Morphologic, cytogenetic, cell surface and enzymatic properties of cultures derived from splenic tumours. *J. Exp. Med.*, **145**, 1484.

5. Curran, R. C. and Jones, E. L. (1977). Hodgkin's disease: an immunohistochemical and histological study. *J. Pathol.*, **125**, 39.

6. Lukes, R. J. and Butler, J. J. (1966). The pathology and nomenclature of Hodgkin's disease. *Cancer Res.* **26** (Part 1), 1063.

7. Lukes, R. J., Craver, L. F., Hall, T. C., Rappaport, H. and Rubin, P. (1966). Report of the Nomenclature Committee. *Cancer Res.*, **26** (Part 1), 1311.

8. Lukes, R. J. (1971). Criteria for involvement of lymph node, bone marrow, spleen and liver in Hodgkin's disease. *Cancer Res.*, **31**, 1755.

9. Lukes, R. J., Tindle, B. H. and Parker, J. W. (1969). Reed–Sternberg-like cells in infectious mononucleosis. (Letter). *Lancet*, **2**, 1003.

10. Strum, S. B., Park, J. K. and Rappaport, H. (1970). Observations of cells resembling Sternberg–Reed cells in conditions other than Hodgkin's disease. *Cancer*, **26**, 176.

11. Kadin, M. E., Glatstein, E. and Dorfman, R. F. (1970). Isolated granulomas in Hodgkin's disease. *N. Engl. J. Med.*, **283**, 859.

12. Kadin, M. E., Glatstein, E. and Dorfman, R. F. (1971). Clinicopathologic studies of 117 untreated patients subjected to laparotomy for the staging of Hodgkin's disease. *Cancer*, **27**, 1277.

Non-Hodgkin's Lymphoma

12

Introduction

This negative form of nomenclature is one of con-
venience. Of the total number of lymphomas,
approximately 40% can be separated under the
general heading of Hodgkin's disease, leaving the
remainder, a conglomerate of very different conditions. Some at least are readily distinguishable
from the rest, but new entities are still in the
process of recognition and description. There is at
present no universally accepted method of classification and whichever system is adopted, a
certain number of tumours defy classification
altogether.

Clearly, any logical classification of lymphomas
should be based on the cell of origin, as is done with
other types of neoplasia. It is only following
relatively recent advances in the field of immunology,
that the function of lymph nodes has begun to be
understood, together with appreciation of the considerable cytological changes which cells of the
immune system can undergo in the expression of
their normal role. This has provided the basis for
modern methods of classification, enabling types of
neoplastic proliferation to be both predicted and
recognized.

More than one group of workers have suggested
classifications with a functional basis, foremost
among them being Lennert[1] in Germany and Lukes
and Collins[2, 3] in the United States. These, and
many others[4], have carried out painstaking investigations involving the study of cell surface
characteristics, cell culture, cytochemistry and
electron microscopy. As a result certain lymphomas which can be characterized by these means
have been correlated with distinctive histological
appearances, recognizable on ordinary paraffin
sections.

It is to the latter that this account is almost
exclusively confined, since this is the universal
experience, but, in doing so, it is acknowledged that
interpretation is based on the specialist studies
undertaken so laboriously by others. It will be seen
that in some cases firm functional parallels cannot
be drawn and then classification must rest upon a
careful evaluation of cytological features.

The essential problems in the field of the non-
Hodgkin's lymphomas are as follows. First, that
although there is a large measure of agreement in
principle as the theoretical basis for classification,
there is not complete agreement as to terminology,
making it difficult to distill a clear concept available
to pathologists at large. Secondly, that having a
functional basis for classification is not enough:
clear histopathological guidelines are required in
order to insert lymphomas as they are actually
encountered, i.e. as histological appearances, into
their appropriate place in the classification. In
addition, such guidelines need to be as simple and
clear as possible, in order to achieve some
uniformity of classification, otherwise there is
little hope of real progress in correlating the clinical
and therapeutic aspects. Lastly, in relation to this,
clinicians on the whole are little interested in
surface markers and transformation of lymphocytes,
since their concern is with their patients, and they
require information relevant to prognosis and
treatment.

Therefore the ideal classification would combine
both theoretical and practical aspects, but in
practice some form of compromise has to be
adopted. The results of the National Lymphoma
Investigation Trials in Great Britain are being
expressed in the working classification of Henry,
Bennett and Farrer-Brown[5] who offer clinicians
two broad grades of malignancy as a therapeutic
guide. Although no longer acceptable for theoretical
reasons, the original concept of Rappaport[6] is still
warmly supported by clinicians[7], who can both
understand it and find within it clinical applications.

The account given here of classification is in no
way original. It uses the terminology of Lukes and
Collins for the follicular centre cells, that of 'cleaved'
and 'uncleaved', acknowledging that many 'cleaved'
cells in fact have only irregular nuclei and often as
not there are extrusions from the nuclear membrane
rather than notches. The advantages of their terms
are that they are simple, call to mind an image and
lastly are unprejudiced, so that they will not
conflict with advances in understanding of function
which may occur in the future.

Therefore, the overall approach to classification
adopted here is dichotomous. On the one hand
awareness of normal cells and their development
suggests stages at which neoplasia could arise.
On the other, there is an attempt to rationalize the
morphological appearances of lymphomas, as
actually encountered. The assessment of any
particular case requires a combination of both
viewpoints.

The analysis of the histological appearance of
a lymphoma is similar to that applied to any other
neoplasm. First, any semblance of pattern is sought,
to enable the basic division to be made between
those of follicular or nodular nature and those which
are diffuse. Further subdivision depends upon a
detailed cytological assessment.

Amongst the diffuse lymphomas there are those
whose overall appearance is varied or heterogeneous. This may result from variations in a single
cell type or may be due to a mixture of cell types.
Other lymphomas have a uniform or homogeneous

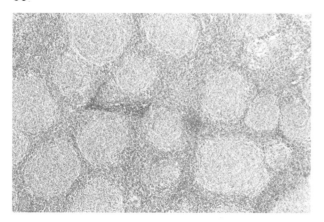

Figure 12.1 A lymphoma of obvious follicular pattern, derived from follicular centre cells. H & E × 36.5.

Figure 12.2 Although this is essentially a diffuse lymphoma, there is fine compartmentalization with collagen fibres present throughout. The cells composing it approximate closest to small cleaved follicular centre cells, but tend to have less nuclear irregularity. This lymphoma presented as generalised lymphadenopathy in a 36-year-old man who is well eight years later. H & E × 36.5.

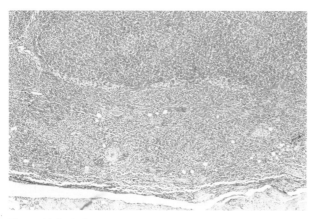

Figure 12.3 Diffuse small cell lymphoma in a patient with the clinical syndrome of Waldenström's macroglobulinaemia. There is extensive capsular infiltration. H & E × 36.5.

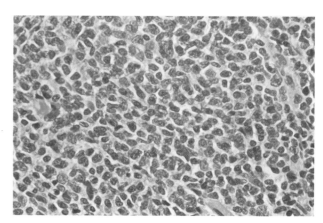

Figure 12.4 Monotony in the small cleaved follicular centre cell population differentiates the neoplastic follicle from a reactive centre. H & E × 365.

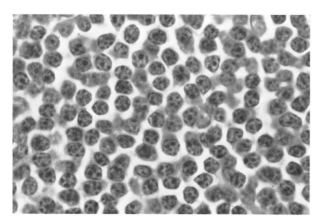

Figure 12.5 Lymphocytic lymphoma. The uniform population of small lymphocytes closely resembles its normal counterpart. H & E × 910

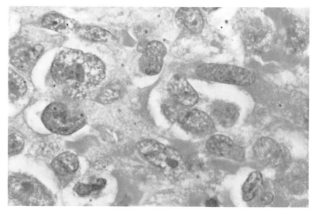

Figure 12.6 A large cell lymphoma, probably histiocytic in type. The cell nuclei tend to be elongated with convex outlines and nucleoli are small but distinct. The pale eosinophilic cytoplasm is abundant. H & E × 910

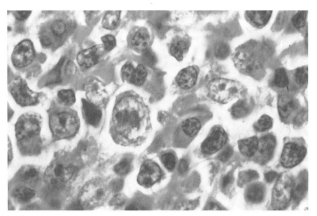

Figure 12.7 The largest cell in this field is an immunoblast with slightly shrunken cytoplasm. Near it is a mature plasma cell. Other cells in the field are intermediate in size between the two and illustrate one possible source from which lymphomas composed of medium sized cells could arise. H & E ×910

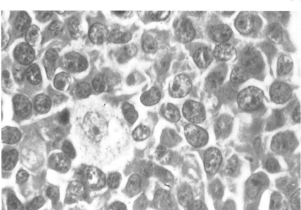

Figure 12.8 Lymphoblastic lymphoma or lymphoma of medium sized lymphoid cells. The axillary node from a young woman showed a histological resemblance to Burkitt's lymphoma. It also contained what appeared to be giant follicular centres with numerous macrophages when examined at low-power, but these too showed the same cytological features as the diffuse lymphoma present elsewhere. H & E ×910.

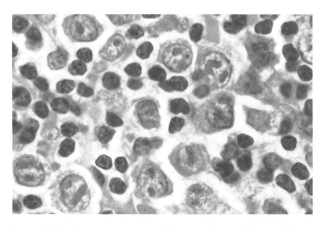

Figure 12.9 Reactive paracortex with immunoblasts. H & E ×910.

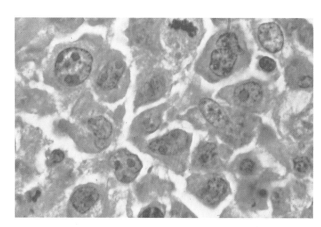

Figure 12.10 Large cell lymphoma. Cytologically the term immunoblastic is appropriate. H & E ×910.

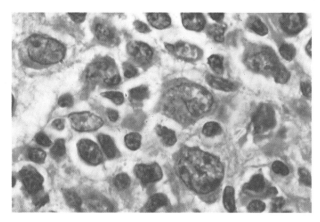

Figure 12.11 'Mixed' or 'mixed cell' lymphoma. Small irregular lymphoid cells interspersed with large cells, in the more open nuclei of which, distinct nucleoli are easily seen. H & E ×910.

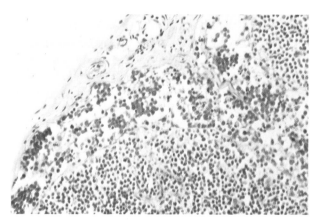

Figure 12.12 Spread of non-Hodgkin's lymphoma. Lymph nodes adjacent to a lymphoblastic lymphoma show invasion of the marginal sinus by neoplastic cells. H & E ×91.

appearance, being composed of cells similar in size and type. This group can be further subdivided using the arbitrary criterion of cell size. The criterion is applied by comparing the size of the predominant neoplastic cells with normal cells in the same tissue, although the lymphomatous population cannot be expected to be entirely monomorphous (see page 64).

Approximate groupings can therefore be made and, in practice, these prove useful. 'Small cell' lymphomas are composed of cells approximating in size to that of small lymphocytes. The nuclei of cells in 'large cell' lymphomas are at least the same size or larger than histiocytic nuclei. Between these two groups are lymphomas composed predominantly of cells of medium or intermediate size. Although at the upper end this latter group includes tumours whose cell nuclei also approximate in size to the nuclei of histiocytes, their characteristic overall appearance (see Burkitt's lymphoma, page 74) means that they are unlikely to be confused with large cell lymphomas in practice.

Functional Basis of Classification

Outline

The outline of the scheme is indicated in the diagram (Plate IV). Essentially, the precursor cells are either B or T lymphocytes or histiocytes. But some lymphomas are composed of cells having no surface markers at all. Lukes and Collins[2] refer to these as null cells. Although lack of recognizable surface characteristics may be due entirely to the primitive nature of the cells in certain proliferations, it is not inconceivable that there are a few precursor cells with the same characteristics in normal tissues.

The diagram gives some points as to possible pathways and potential sites for neoplastic transformation. It indicates the source of the numerically important follicular lymphomas and the explanation for the cytological variation that occurs within the group. Possible further B lymphocyte pathways of development are also indicated.

B Lymphocytes as Precursor Cells

By far the majority of non-Hodgkin's lymphomas derive from the B lymphocyte population and, as might have been predicted, it is the sites of active proliferation, the follicular centres, which contribute the greatest proportion. The distinguishing feature of this group is that cellular expansion is not entirely random. To some extent, follicular arrangement is maintained and it is for this reason, as well as the cytological relationships with their normal counterparts, that these form a well-defined group and are separated from the rest of the non-Hodgkin's lymphomas, which are therefore referred to as diffuse.

Lukes and Collins[2] have also suggested that another contribution is made by follicular centres, in the form of true Burkitt's lymphoma and related types. They are of the opinion that the proliferating cell in these conditions is the small non-cleaved follicular centre cell.

Both before and after their passage through the follicular centres, the B lymphocytes can have the morphological appearance associated with normal small lymphocytes. Proliferations resulting from these precursor cells give rise to lymph nodes identical in appearance to those in chronic lymphocytic leukaemia. The extremely close relationship between the conditions can be appreciated by imagining the neoplastic change intervening either in lymphocytes still in the bone marrow or perhaps just a little later in development where they have reached the lymph nodes, and either await entry into the follicular centres, or have passed through them. Berard et al.[8] have shown that the majority of small lymphocytes in cases of chronic lymphocytic leukaemia and lymphocytic lymphoma bear scanty IgM. Lymphocytes with similar characteristics are found in the medullary cords of normal nodes and, in the absence of further development in the node itself, these leave in the efferent lymph. It is not therefore surprising that many cases of lymphocytic lymphoma, defined initially because of the proliferation taking place principally in the lymph nodes rather than the bone marrow, subsequently change over to a leukaemic phase indistinguishable from cases which are leukaemic from the outset.

There may or may not be secretory activity on the part of the neoplastic B lymphocytes but when this occurs, the finding of abnormal proteins in the serum is usually accompanied by evidence of plasmacytoid differentiation in the cells. One example is Waldenström's macroglobulinaemia, where there is not only IgM on the surface of the cell but it is also secreted into the extracellular environment. But other classes of immunoglobulin may also be secreted by neoplastic B cells.

In normal reactive nodes foci of apparent plasma cell proliferation can be recognized, with primitive-looking large cells associated with others more recognizable as having plasma cell characteristics. Perhaps these are areas of clonal expansion. This substrate provides for a variety of B cell lymphomas, and in particular could be the source of some of the large cell lymphomas, which may or may not give evidence of their origin. In states of prolonged and abnormal B cell proliferation, for instance autoimmune disorders, when neoplastic transformation occurs, it is often in the form of this large cell lymphoma. Where the antecedents are clear, Lukes has suggested that the term 'immunoblastic sarcoma' is appropriate.

Many of the lymphomas composed of medium-sized cells, the lymphoblastic lymphomas, also derive from different stages of B lymphocyte development and it is difficult to pinpoint precisely the stages at which all of these arise.

Lastly, there are tumours composed of mature plasma cells, primary extra-medullary plasmacytomas. Whilst not so rare as formerly thought, they are still uncommon in lymph nodes although more frequently recognized in extra-nodal sites. This suggests that mature plasma cells as such are relatively resistant to neoplastic transformation, and that there is some special factor in the environment of the bone marrow, or that they are peculiarly vulnerable during their development in that site.

T Lymphocytes as Precursor Cells

The contribution that T lymphocytes make towards lymphomas is relatively restricted. They form a small number of lymphocytic lymphomas (as they do of cases of chronic lymphocytic leukaemia), presumably some lymphomas of medium-sized cells, and certainly contribute to the undifferentiated large cell lymphomas, where again the designation 'immunoblastic sarcoma' could be applied. There is however, on histological grounds alone, no way of distinguishing these T cell neoplasms. They lack the tell-tale cytological changes associated with the secretory activity of the B lymphocytes.

Therefore, only those tumours with histological features which can be associated with a T lymphocyte pedigree can be recognized as separate entities. Interesting in this regard, is the lymphoma arising from nodal T lymphocytes, which is well described by Waldron et al.[9], in which the proliferating lymphoid cells are intimately mixed with non-neoplastic histiocytes. This is an intriguing observation, in that it suggests the possibility of lymphokine production by the neoplastic cells, and perhaps parallels will be recognized in other situations.

Another example of T lymphocyte neoplasia is that which occurs apparently during the phase of development within the thymus. Most of these tumours develop in young boys, and the characteristic, rather irregular, neoplastic cells have been referred to as convoluted cells, this term being used in the name, convoluted cell lymphoma.

This feature of convolution of nuclear outline seems to be associated with T lymphocytes, and the condition reaches its zenith in the neoplastic proliferations which are generated from the T lymphocytes associated with the skin. In mycosis fungoides, lymph nodes can become extensively replaced by the lymphoid cells peculiar to this condition, and even deep tissues remote from the sites of skin involvement may also be infiltrated. In the allied state of Sezary's syndrome, even greater nuclear convolution characterizes the cells and this has been demonstrated particularly well by electron microscopy, (Lutzner et al.[10]).

Histiocytes as Precursor Cells

In discussing the proliferations of histiocytic cells, we are looking at a whole spectrum of behaviour, in terms of differentiation and aggression. To some extent, an arbitrary line has to be drawn between those conditions in which there is restraint, the histiocytoses; and those which are unequivocally malignant. In the latter category are the conditions of histiocytic lymphoma (a term which is acceptable, if lymphoma be interpreted as a tumour of lymph nodes, rather than lymphoid cells) and malignant histiocytosis.

Histiocytic lymphoma can present in three guises. First, it contributes to the class of large cell lymphomas where there is no evidence of differentiation. Secondly, in a few rare cases, the cells very much resemble normal histiocytes and occasionally even show phagocytosis. Lastly, an extremely unusual group of tumours, where many of the cells seem to have features of histiocytes, but the appearance overall is bizarre because a number of the nuclei are extremely large, irregular and dense. This has been aptly described as a pleomorphic histiocytic lymphoma[6].

Malignant histiocytosis is a systemic disorder and is discussed under the heading of histiocytoses (Chapter 16); the neoplastic histiocytes are confined initially within the sinuses, where they may show considerable evidence of function, but finally the pulp of the node is invaded and, in some cases, the original sinus origin may be unrecognizable, making the appearance indistinguishable from a histiocytic lymphoma.

Null Cells as Precursors

On balance this category of cells is probably too primitive in nature to express surface characteristics. A third of large cell lymphomas lack identifiable markers (Berard et al.[8]), as do a number of the acute lymphoblastic leukaemias.

Morphological Approach to Classification

Pattern

Lymphomas exhibiting a follicular pattern are separated from the rest which are termed diffuse. The diffuse lymphomas have a fairly uniform overall appearance, because the majority of neoplastic cells conform to a certain size range and can be grouped on the basis of size of the predominant cell. Alternatively, diffuse lymphomas may have a variable histological appearance, due to differences in cell size and/or cell type in their composition.

Follicular Lymphomas

These arise from follicular centre cells and cleaved cells (small or large) or non-cleaved cells may predominate. Alternatively, there may be a mixture of these cell types. (Diffuse lymphomas of similar cytological composition also occur.)

Diffuse Lymphomas of Homogeneous Appearance

(a) *Small cells predominate*
Lymphocytic lymphoma (chronic lymphocytic leukaemia)
Small lymphocytes with plasmacytoid differentiation (commonly associated with IgM production).
Small cells with irregular nuclei (resemble small cleaved follicular centre cells but no evidence of pre-existing follicular pattern).

(b) *Medium size cells predominate*
Burkitt's lymphoma (? derived from follicular centre cells).
Lymphomas bearing a close histological resemblance to Burkitt's lymphoma.
Lymphoblastic lymphoma (with or without plasmacytoid differentiation).
Extra-medullary plasmacytoma (mature plasma cells).
Lymphoblastic lymphoma of convoluted cell type.
(Acute lymphoblastic leukaemia)

(c) *Large cells predominate*
Large non-cleaved follicular centre cells.
Large cleaved follicular centre cells.
Immunoblastic lymphoma.
Histiocytic lymphoma.
Large cell lymphoma, unspecified.
(Acute granulocytic leukaemias).

Diffuse Lymphomas of Heterogeneous Appearance

Mixed follicular centre cells.
Pleomorphic histiocytic lymphoma.
Pleomorphic plasmacytoid lymphoma.

Lymphoma arising from peripheral T lymphocytes.

Malignant lymphoma with a high content of epithelioid histiocytes.

(Mycosis fungoides).

Presence of Sclerosis in Non-Hodgkin's Lymphomas

Sclerosis does not appear to play such a conspicuous and important role as it does in Hodgkin's disease. However Bennett's analysis[11] of over 200 cases suggests that its presence is significant, leading to a slightly improved prognosis.

In assessing fibrosis, apparently stimulated by the presence of neoplastic cells, it is necessary to decide whether it was likely to have been pre-existing. This is self-evident in nodes from the inguinal region, but the frequency of fibrosis occurring in nodes from the mesentery and retro-peritoneum is referred to by Rosas-Uribe and Rappaport[12].

Two principal patterns of fibrosis are to be distinguished. One is the presence of broad fibrous bands, especially in follicular lymphomas, where they separate the nodules. Bennett[11] found that over a third of his cases of follicular lymphoma exhibited this feature in some degree, but the proportion of our cases in which it has provoked comment is much lower.

The other pattern is that of what appears to be a reticulin network, separating groups of cells, and referred to as compartmentalizing fibrosis by Rosas-Uribe and Rappaport[12]. This is seen particularly in various of the large cell lymphomas, and the apparent 'nests' of cells may lead to an incorrect diagnosis of carcinoma.

In addition fibrosis develops following therapy, when both patterns described above, as well as more diffuse sclerotic change can occur. Prognostic significance can only be attached to the initial biopsy, and seems to be most accentuated with regard to the follicular lymphomas.

Granulomas in Non-Hodgkin's Lymphoma

Whilst epithelioid granulomas are not infrequent in association with Hodgkin's disease, and may be very conspicuous indeed in some cases, they are not a common accompaniment of the non-Hodgkin's lymphomas. Dorfman and Kim[13] reported sarcoid-like granulomas both in lymph nodes and other tissues, but make the point that their presence should not influence staging procedures. At the present time their significance is not understood, but they seem to have no prognostic implications.

Prognosis in Non-Hodgkin's Lymphoma

The possible favourable influence of the presence of sclerosis has already been mentioned and the question of follicular pattern is discussed in Chapter 13. Apart from these two considerations, categorizing lymphomas on the basis of predominant cell size is itself of prognostic value. Small cell lymphomas are only slowly progressive whilst those composed of medium sized or large cells behave as aggressive tumours. This is despite the fact that many small cell lymphomas are already widespread at presentation, a finding probably explicable by the tendency of their

normal cell counterparts to circulate.

But Taylor[14], discussing mainly B lymphocytes, has once more drawn attention to the stages of development of normal cells and the morphological changes associated with the cell cycle. He has stressed the polymorphous nature of monoclonal proliferations. When these are studied, the emphasis is usually put upon the more mature elements to aid identification of the precursor cell type, but more attention should be paid to the less mature cells which represent the proliferative component. This is after all the practice in assessing leukaemias and non-lymphoid neoplasms.

Two implications arise out of appreciation that the lymphomatous population includes an active proliferating compartment of immature cells. The first is that there may be a dramatic change in the nature of any lymphoma or leukaemia, due to a sudden increase in the number of immature cells. This process is sometimes referred to as transmutation. The other is more subtle and should be applied to the histological assessment of any individual case. Some comment should be made upon the proportion of large cells present, because this can vary within each separate category of classification, no matter which system is preferred. Not only does this give a more accurate guide to prognosis but enables appropriate treatment to be directed against disease which is becoming more aggressive. Thus, a small cell lymphoma with a significant proportion of large cells must be expected to behave differently from one containing very few large cells.

Further study is necessary to elucidate the significance of reactive cells in non-Hodgkin's lymphoma. Their presence could indicate host response, as in Hodgkin's disease, or be evidence of maturity and function on the part of neoplastic cells themselves (see page 63). Either of these possibilities could be of prognostic importance.

References

1. Lennert, K., Stein, H. and Kaiserling, E. (1975). Cytological and functional criteria for the classification of the malignant lymphomata. Symposium on non-Hodgkin's lymphomata. *Br. J. Cancer*, **31** (Suppl. 2), 29.

2. Lukes, R. J. and Collins, R. D. (1975). New approaches to the classification of the lymphomata. Symposium on non-Hodgkin's lymphomata. *Br. J. Cancer*, **31** (Suppl. II), 1.

3. Lukes, R. J. and Collins, R. D. (1974). New approaches to the classification of malignant lymphomas. *Cancer*, **34**, 1488.

4. Jaffe, E. S., Shevach, E. M., Frank, M. M., Berard, C. W. and Green, I. (1974). Nodular lymphoma — evidence for origin from follicular B lymphocytes. *N. Engl. J. Med.*, **290**, 813.

5. Henry, K., Bennett, M. H. and Farrer-Brown, G. (1978). Classification of the non-Hodgkin's lymphomas. In P. P. Anthony and N. Woolf (eds.) *Recent Advances in Histopathology*, pp. 275-302, (Churchill Livingstone).

6. Rappaport, H. (1966). *Tumors of the Haematopoietic System*. Atlas of Tumor Pathology — Section III — Fascicle 8. (Washington, D.C.: Armed Forces Institute of Pathology).

7. Portlock, C. S. and Glatstein, E. (1978). The non-Hodgkin's lymphomas: current concepts and management. *Ann. Rev. Med.*, **29**, 81.

8. Berard, C. W., Jaffe, E. S., Braylan, R. C., Mann, R. B. and Nanba, K. (1978). Immunological aspects and pathology of the malignant lymphomas. *Cancer*, **42**, 911.

9. Waldron, J. A., Leech, J. H., Glick, A. D., Flexner, J. M. and Collins, R. D. (1977). Malignant lymphoma of peripheral T-lymphocyte origin. *Cancer*, **40**, 1604.

10. Lutzner, M. A., Hobbs, J. W. and Horvath, P. (1971). Ultrastructure of abnormal cells in Sezary syndrome, mycosis fungoides and parapsoriasis en plaque. *Arch. Dermatol.*, **103**, 375.
11. Bennett, M. H. (1975). Sclerosis in non-Hodgkin's lymphomata. *Br. J. Cancer*, **31** (Suppl. 2), 44.
12. Rosas-Uribe, A. and Rappaport, H. (1972). Malignant lymphoma histiocytic type with sclerosis (sclerosing reticulum cell sarcoma). *Cancer*, **29**, 946.
13. Dorfman, R. F. and Kim, H. (1975). Relationship of histology to site in the non-Hodgkin's lymphomata. A study based on surgical staging procedures. *Br. J. Cancer*, **31** (Suppl. 2), 217.
14. Taylor, C. R. (1978). Classification of lymphoma. 'New thinking' on old thoughts. *Arch. Pathol. Lab. Med.*, **102**, 549.

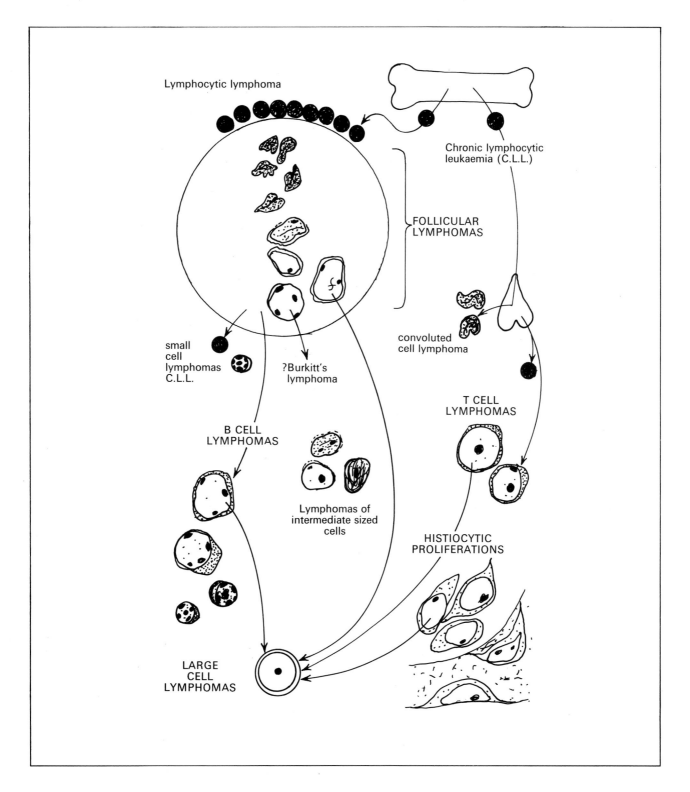

Plate IV Some potential sources of non-Hodgkins lymphomas.

Follicular Centre Cell Lymphomas (Follicular Lymphomas)

13

Introduction

The majority of non-Hodgkin's lymphomas are follicular in pattern and are thought to arise from the cells of the follicular or germinal centres. Initially this view was based upon cytological correlations which exist between neoplastic and reactive follicular structures but in addition, the cells of follicular lymphomas have been demonstrated to have the surface marker characteristics of B lymphocytes. Further, at ultrastructural level, the presence of dendritic reticular cells can be demonstated within neoplastic follicles, just as in reactive centres.

Cytological Features

The variable appearance of cells found within normal reactive centres has been referred to already (see page 15), but the features are indicated again in Plate IV. Thus there are small and large forms of 'cleaved' cell, with peculiar nuclear irregularities (deep notches, folds or extrusions of the nuclear membrane) and rather insignificant cytoplasm (Figures 13.6, 13.7). These contrast with the 'non-cleaved' cells whose nuclei are vesicular, rounded in outline, contain small but distinct nucleoli, often close to the nuclear membrane and have a moderate amount of amphophilic cytoplasm (Figure 13.9). The non-cleaved cells also are not uniform in size and can be conveniently described as 'small' and 'large'.

These differing appearances presumably represent stages in the development of the lymphoid cells within the follicular centres. It seems reasonable to assume that neoplastic proliferation could be initiated at those different stages of development and that the resulting tumours would be composed of the cell type appropriate to that stage. The assumption appears to be at least partially correct. Often it is a single follicular centre cell type which predominates in the neoplastic follicles. It may be virtually exclusive and it is this which imparts the characteristic monotonous appearance which is such a useful diagnostic feature (Figure 12.4).

Thus, neoplastic follicles composed predominantly of cleaved or non-cleaved cells occur, but in some cases the cell population is a mixed one. Quite apart from the nature of the neoplastic cells present at the time of presentation, there is ample evidence of a change in cytological composition, during the course of the disease in some patients. This can be seen in sequential biopsies or sometimes illustrated in a single biopsy. The pattern of progression which takes place involves a change from a predominantly small cleaved cell population towards a predominantly large, non-cleaved cell neoplasm (Figure 13.9). At times, only occasional large non-cleaved cells may be present, but they appear to increase gradually or form definite foci. Finally, although this may take several years to develop, it appears that the large non-cleaved component becomes dominant and this has been referred to as 'malignant transformation' of a follicular lymphoma, since the indolent phase of its behaviour is over.

The mitotic rate, as it appears upon histological examination, amongst follicular lymphomas of small cleaved cell type is variable. It can be either very low indeed or moderately conspicuous. The mitotic rate seen in large non-cleaved cell tumours is moderate or high.

Follicular Pattern

There are some correlations between the cytological features and the follicular pattern of these lymphomas. The degree of retention of a follicular arrangement presumably represents the extent to which the organization of the neoplasm reproduces normal reactive follicular formation. With progression of the lymphoma, the follicular structures become less well defined and as their edges become blurred (Figure 13.2), they are usually much larger. As this change takes place, the focal character may disappear altogether and the lymphoma is then described as diffuse.

Therefore, well marked follicular arrangement is often associated with proliferations of the small cleaved cell type. As the larger cell component increases in the population, this is linked with gradual loss of follicular pattern in most cases, so that by the time the large non-cleaved cells have become pre-eminent, the nature of the proliferation is entirely diffuse.

A reticulin stained section is essential in that it accentuates the follicular nature, since the neoplastic foci expand at the expense of the pre-existing tissue and compress the fibre framework (Figure 9.3).

Recognition of an early follicular lymphoma is often difficult. There may be a surrounding mantle of small lymphocytes (Figure 9.1), so that a normal reactive centre is closely mimicked and in the early stages there may still be reactive follicular centres present in the node, confusing interpretation even further. Where neoplastic follicles are still confined within the node, distinction rests upon a careful evaluation of the cytological features. The replacement of normal functional zones by follicular structures without accompanying plasma cell increase, may be a helpful adjunct. Once the

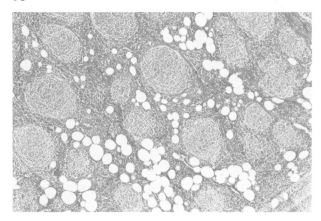

Figure 13.1 Maintenance of follicular pattern of proliferation as adipose tissue is invaded. H & E ×36.5.

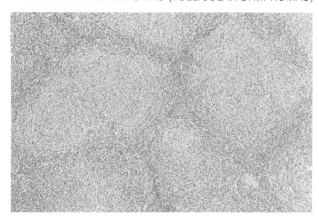

Figure 13.2 Follicular centre cell lymphoma. Follicular pattern is still present but there is blurring of the edges of follicular structures. No lymphocyte mantle is present. H & E ×36.5.

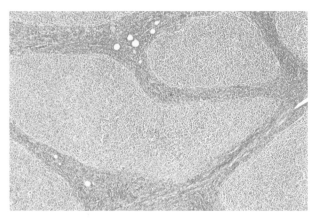

Figure 13.3 Follicular centre cell lymphoma. Neoplastic follicles are not always round and uniform in size. Like reactive follicles they can be greatly elongated or bizarre in shape (see also Figure 9.2). H & E ×36.5.

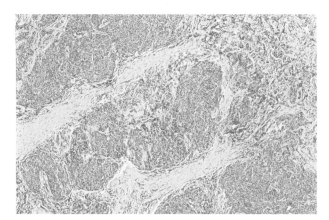

Figure 13.4 Follicular centre cell lymphoma. Well marked bands of sclerosis are present. H & E ×36.5.

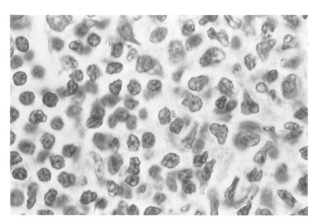

Figure 13.5 Follicular centre cell lymphoma. The contrast between small lymphocytes and the small cleaved cells of the lymphoma is demonstrated at the edge of a neoplastic follicle. H & E ×910.

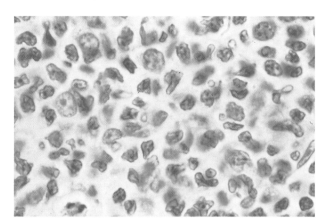

Figure 13.6 Follicular centre cell lymphoma. Predominantly small cleaved cells but an occasional larger rounded nucleus is present. H & E ×910.

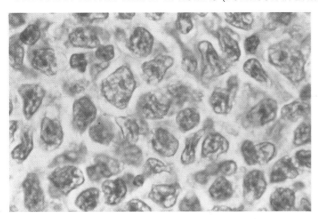

Figure 13.7 Follicular centre cell lymphoma. Predominantly large cleaved cells. H & E ×910.

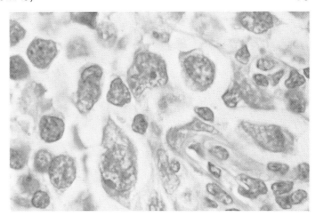

Figure 13.8 Follicular centre cell lymphoma. The appearance of a biopsy four years after the first lymph node examination had shown a predominantly small cleaved cell population, as Figure 13.6. The presence of large cells now gives a much more mixed cytological appearance. H & E ×910.

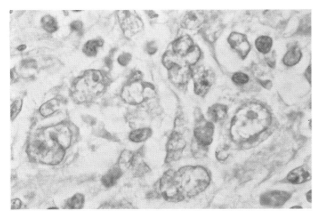

Figure 13.9 In another patient, eight years after diagnosis of a well defined follicular lymphoma composed almost exclusively of small cleaved cells, sudden localized nodal enlargement occurred. Diffuse lymphoma composed of large non-cleaved cells was present in a second biopsy. H & E ×910.

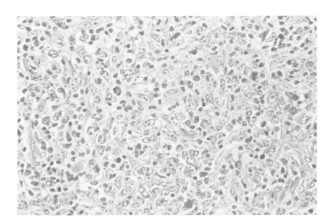

Figure 13.10 (From the same case as Figure 13.9). This illustrates the diffuse nature of the large cell lymphoma which developed. It appeared to extend from a previous obviously follicular area, composed of small cleaved cells. H & E ×230.

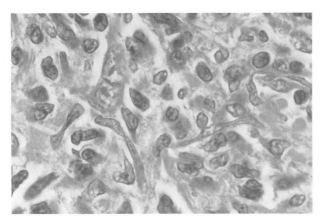

Figure 13.11 Follicular centre cell lymphoma. Bizarre elongated nuclei within follicular structures suggest considerable cell motility. The largest cell could represent a dendritic reticular cell. H & E ×910.

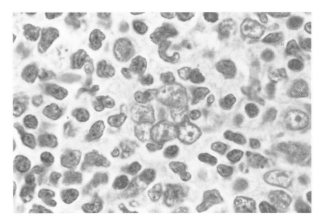

Figure 13.12 Follicular centre cell lymphoma. Mulberry-like clusters of nuclei can be observed not infrequently. The impression is that they represent multinucleated cells, rather than a close group of single cells. The nuclei are usually open and small distinct nucleoli are present. H & E ×910.

lymphoma extends beyond the capsule or into adipose tissue in the central part of the node, the neoplastic nature of the follicular proliferation may be clearly recognized (Figure 13.1).

Other Features

The number of phagocytic macrophages within neoplastic follicles is extremely variable. Occasionally they are present in moderate numbers but in about half the cases they are entirely absent. This is particularly true with regard to the small cleaved cell type, where little occurs to disturb the monotonous appearance.

In the behaviour of the small cleaved cell type there is an apparent anomaly. As stated above, follicular pattern is well maintained and yet at the same time there can be extensive seeding of the characteristic neoplastic cells through the tissues, away from the apparent focus of disease. The cells can be recognized in the 'interfollicular' areas, in the lymph sinuses, and frequently in the bone marrow. Often, their 'cleaved' nature is less accentuated in these extra-follicular sites, their nuclei appearing rather smaller and less irregular. It is possible therefore in this particular class of lymphoma to have a patient at an advanced stage of the disease with regard to its widespread nature and yet to be quite well, with a relatively indolent condition and reasonable prognosis.

Occasionally, in lymphomas of small cleaved cell type, there are large cells containing a cluster of nuclei (Figure 13.12). Several of these cells may be close together in a focal area. The nuclei are round to oval, rather larger than those of small lymphocytes and have a distinct nucleolus. They may contain moderate chromatin, or be rather empty, and not unlike histiocyte nuclei. These multinucleate cells are reminiscent of those seen in some virus infections. At the light microscope level, it seems reasonable to postulate that they are derived from dendritic reticular cells. If so, it may eventually be shown that follicular lymphomas develop as a result of abnormality in the dendritic reticular cells, rather than a direct effect of some agent on the follicular centre cells themselves.

Another histological feature of variable incidence is the presence of eosinophilic, amorphous material deposited within neoplastic follicles, exactly as can be seen in normal lymphoid tissue, especially in the spleen. Attention was drawn to this deposited material by Rosas-Uribe et al.[1], and besides showing its diastase-resistant PAS positivity, they found it had a fibrillary structure, and was associated with desmosomes, when viewed ultrastructurally. It seems entirely likely that this is material associated with the surface of dendritic reticular cells and may well include antigen–antibody complexes. Its presence has no significance in terms of behaviour of any given follicular lymphoma.

Prognosis in Follicular Lymphoma

Prognosis is to be related both to the cytology of the proliferation and to the extent to which follicular pattern is maintained. As already stated, these appear to be interrelated. Curiously enough, the extent of the disease at the time of presentation is less important; it seems to reflect the fact that the aggressiveness of the disease process rests more in the proliferative activity of the cells than in their widespread dispersal through tissues, which probably only reflects some aspect of normal biological behaviour. Indeed, it may be better to view this early widespread involvement by small cleaved cells, simply as a 'spill-over' phenomenon, assuming that their normal progression through the follicular centre stage of development is blocked. This can be contrasted with the rapid proliferation of large non-cleaved follicular centre cells, which behave as an aggressive, poorly differentiated neoplasm, even though fairly localized at onset.

Clearly, the cytological evaluation has important prognostic implications and whilst at the two ends of the spectrum there is little difficulty, there are many cases which fall in between and contain a mixture of cell types. Lukes and Collins[2], after an analysis of their own cases, have suggested that where the cell population shows areas of focal dominance by large non-cleaved cells, or where they contribute about 25% of the total, then the patient should be classified as having a follicular lymphoma of non-cleaved cell type. Such a histological appearance implies evolution to the aggressive form of the disease, and in practice it makes little difference whether the large non-cleaved cells contribute a quarter, or the whole population.

Similarly, the presence of large non-cleaved cells overrides the other factor of prognostic significance, the retention of follicular pattern. Where this is present in the other cytological types, it does seem to indicate a better overall prognosis[3], even when combined with diffuse areas[4], but has no effect at all where non-cleaved cells contribute 25% or more of the population.

References

1. Rosas-Uribe, A., Variakojis, D. and Rappaport, H. (1973). Proteinaceous precipitate in nodular (follicular) lymphomas. *Cancer*, **31**, 534.
2. Lukes, R. J. and Collins, R. D. (1975). New approaches to the classification of the lymphomata. *Br. J. Cancer*, **31** (Suppl. 2), 1.
3. Butler, J. J., Stryker, J. A. and Schullenberger, C. C. (1974). A clinico-pathological study of stages I and II non-Hodgkin's lymphomata, using the Lukes-Collins classification. *Br. J. Cancer*, **31** (Suppl. 2), 208.
4. Warnke, R. A., Kim, H., Fuks, Z. and Dorfman, R. F. (1977). The coexistence of nodular and diffuse patterns in nodular non-Hodgkin's lymphomas. *Cancer*, **40**, 1229.

14

Diffuse Non-Hodgkin's Lymphoma of Homogeneous Appearance

Predominantly small cell populations

Introduction

Despite the fact that this group frequently exhibits widespread disease at the time of presentation, the rate of progression is usually slow, suggesting that often the patient does not present clinically in the early stages. This compares with the cases of chronic lymphocytic leukaemia, diagnosed incidentally in the pursuit of other diseases.

Lymphocytic Lymphoma

Strong correlations exist with chronic lymphocytic leukaemia in the majority of patients with this condition, multiple lymph node involvement being succeeded by spread to the bone marrow and blood, although this is not invariable[1]. There are in addition a few cases in which the disease is restricted to a single node, or group of nodes, and in these there is no tendency to a leukaemic phase.

Nodal architecture is effaced by densely packed small lymphocytes, closely resembling their normal counterparts, exhibiting very few mitotic figures. Amongst them may be found a varying proportion of larger lymphoid cells showing mitotic activity, which can produce a definite 'pseudofollicular' appearance, when the accumulations are well marked (Figure 14.2). This is referred to again under the heading of chronic lymphocytic leukaemia.

'Macroglobulinaemia' (of Waldenström)

This is a clinical diagnosis, based upon the demonstation of an abnormal band of immunoglobulin in the serum, which is IgM in the majority of cases. The disease usually presents as a result of the abnormality in the serum proteins, but is associated with morphological changes in lymph nodes. Closely akin to lymphocytic lymphoma, which it often resembles, it includes cells which not only have IgM on their surface, but are sufficiently developed to secrete it. Therefore, careful examination reveals a varying number of cells with plasmacytoid features (Figures 14.4 and 14.7).

Again there is no destruction of architecture although the dense infiltration may distort it. Normal features are effaced, but lymphoid follicles may persist for a while and often the sinuses are accentuated, appearing pale because of their histiocyte content[2]. The capsule and surrounding tissues may also show a diffuse infiltration by small cells. Another unexplained feature is that mast cells are moderately frequent, an association that is also seen in non-lymphoid neoplasms.

It must be stressed that, at times, the morphological evidence of secretory activity is only recognized with some difficulty, and the pyronin-methyl-green stain is invaluable in such cases. Whilst not exclusive to macroglobulinaemia, another feature often seen is the presence of intranuclear inclusions of cytoplasm which stain positively by the PAS method and probably represent accumulation of immunoglobulin[3] (Figure 14.5).

In other cases of macroglobulinaemia much more marked and widespread evidence of maturation towards plasma cells is shown and occasionally, in the same clinical syndrome, the nodes show a pseudofollicular pattern with accentuation of plasmacytoid features in the cells between the 'follicular' structures (Figures 14.6–14.8).

Small cleaved cells

Lymphomas of diffuse pattern are encountered in which the predominant cells are regular in size but show the irregular nuclear features associated with the small cleaved follicular centre cells. Usually however the degree of nuclear irregularity is not quite as marked as in follicular lymphomas, and lymphocytes not varying from normal morphology may be admixed[3]. There is no evidence of preceding follicular lymphoma but occasionally a vaguely nodular growth pattern is discernible.

There may be an element of fibrosis with delicate collagen bands present (Figure 12.2). Occasional cells resembling dendritic reticular cells with desmosome junctions have been described in ultrastructural studies suggesting origin from follicular centres. However Berard et al.[4] report finding strong alkaline phosphatase activity at the surface of the proliferating neoplastic lymphocytes. In normal nodes this is shown only by the lymphocytes in primary follicles and the cuffs which surround follicular centres. This observation helps to explain the features which make this a separate entity. At least 10% of these cases have been found to have neoplastic lymphocytes circulating in the blood.

Predominantly large cell populations

The majority of lymphomas included under this heading correspond to the 'reticulum cell sarcomas' of other terminology. Whilst it is not unusual for them to be localized at the outset, their behaviour is usually aggressive and they exhibit rapid progression. This is not, however, invariable in that responses to radical therapy do occur. The factors governing this difference in behaviour are not yet clear although in general terms the presence of reticulin fibres seems to be linked with a better

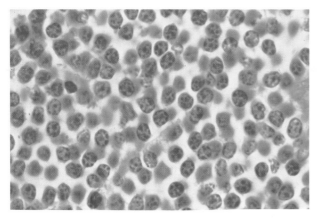

Figure 14.1 Lymphocytic lymphoma. Diffuse replacement of normal lymphoid tissue by uniform cells closely resembling normal small lymphocytes. H & E   ×910.

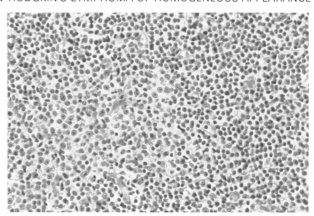

Figure 14.2 Lymphocytic lymphoma. Pseudofollicular appearance of a proliferation centre. H & E   ×230.

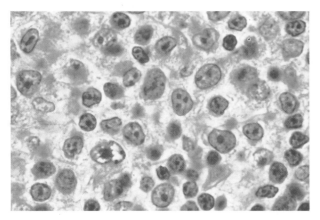

Figure 14.3 Within proliferation centres, medium sized lymphoid cells with round to oval nuclei and distinct nucleoli resemble prolymphocytes, as seen in the bone marrow. These must be interpreted as a component of a small cell lymphoma. H & E   ×910.

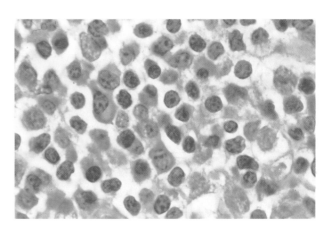

Figure 14.4 Waldenström's macroglobulinaemia. In many patients with this syndrome, the majority of cells resemble normal small lymphocytes. Occasional cells however show definite plasmacytoid features. H & E ×910.

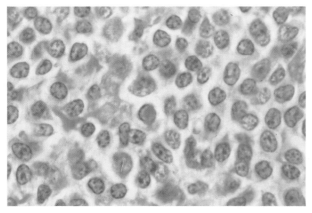

Figure 14.5 In neoplastic proliferations associated with secretion of immunoglobulin, PAS-positive inclusions within the nucleus may be observed. Formed from cytoplasm, they probably contain immunoglobulin. PAS.   ×910

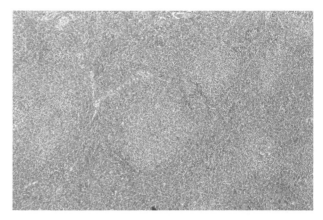

Figure 14.6 A middle-aged man with the clinical syndrome of Waldenström's macroglobulinaemia had a node biopsy performed. The proliferation replacing normal features had a definite nodular pattern. This is not a common finding in association with this syndrome. H & E   ×36.5.

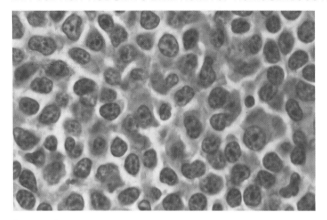

Figure 14.7 (Figures 14.6 to 14.8 are all from the same patient). The nodular areas are composed of cells resembling small lymphocytes, a few of which have a plasmacytoid appearance. Cytologically these areas resemble the common appearance seen in macroglobulinaemia. H & E ×910.

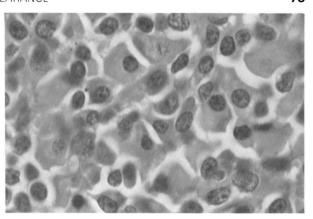

Figure 14.8 In the regions of the node between the 'nodules', almost every cell shows pronounced plasmacytoid features with abundant cytoplasm. H & E ×910.

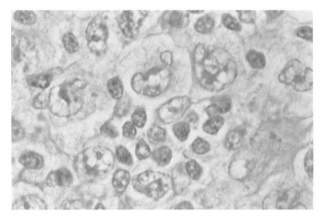

Figure 14.9 Large cell lymphoma. The proliferating cells have open, vesicular nuclei, often oval or reniform in shape, surrounded by extremely abundant, pale eosinophilic cytoplasm. This was interpreted as a histiocytic lymphoma. H & E ×910.

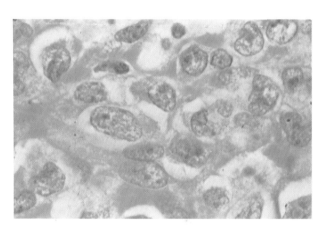

Figure 14.10 Large cell lymphoma. The neoplastic cells again show a considerable resemblance to normal histiocytes. Histiocytic lymphoma. H & E ×910.

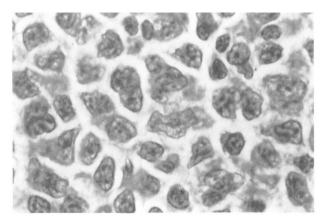

Figure 14.11 Large cell lymphoma composed of cells with angulated, irregular nuclei. Obvious folds in the nuclear membrane are present. Artefactual clear spaces around the nuclei represent shrinkage of cytoplasm. Large cleaved follicular centre cell lymphoma. H & E ×910.

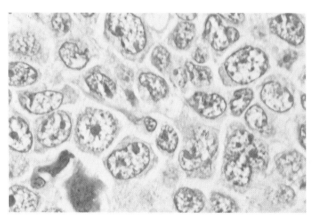

Figure 14.12 Diffuse large cell lymphoma, occurring in an elderly woman without a relevant clinical history. Its source cannot be recognized with certainty but there was a semblance of nodular pattern in one area of the node and the appearance of the cells is compatible with that of large non-cleaved follicular centre cells. H & E ×910.

prognosis. Although this could merely reflect a slower growth rate, it may be the result of some form of cellular activity, indicating a degree of differentiation.

The term 'histiocytic' has also been applied to the class of large cell lymphomas[5] but it is now clear that the majority of them are composed of lymphoid cells. Immunological surface marker studies indicate that 50–60% are of B lymphocyte origin, perhaps 5–10% arise from T lymphocytes and only 5% can be regarded as being truly histiocytic or monocytic in type. The remaining large cell lymphomas lack any demonstrable surface markers at all.

The interpretation of lymphomas in this class, on light microscopy alone, is limited. In some cases, it will be guided by the history. For instance, the previous existence of a follicular centre cell lymphoma argues for final evolution to the diffuse phase, dominated by the large non-cleaved cells. Similarly, disturbed or exaggerated pre-existing B lymphocyte activity predisposes to the emergence of a B immunoblastic sarcoma. In such a case, cells with features of plasmablasts may be present, and the recognition of such changes, even in the absence of a suggestive history, enables a reasonably accurate diagnosis to be made.

Other types of large cell lymphoma which can be distinguished are few. Rarely, the neoplastic cells most resemble the large cleaved cell element of the follicular centres, with irregularity of nuclei and lines in the nuclear membrane, but mostly lacking distinct nucleoli (Figure 14.11). This appearance is not to be confused with true histiocytic lymphoma, also composed of cells with slightly elongated nuclei, where the nuclear membranes are well-defined and nucleoli usually present (Figure 14.9 and 14.10). These cells have a moderate amount of eosinophilic cytoplasm, and occasionally even show phagocytosis. Tumours of such highly differentiated histiocytes are rare. They must in turn be differentiated from the 'spill-over' effect which occurs in malignant histiocytosis (see page 83).

Less differentiated histiocytic neoplasms cannot be diagnosed with confidence, on light microscopy alone. They may however be suspected where the cells have abundant cytoplasm, and the nucleus exhibits a somewhat vesicular appearance, with its outline dominated by rounded protuberances. Another peculiar variant, in which nuclear pleomorphism is the most striking feature, is described in the next Chapter.

Predominantly Medium-sized Cell Populations, 'Lymphoblastic' Lymphoma

Introduction

This group, like its title, lacks precision. Defined as it is in this context, it embraces both recognized entities and other proliferations lacking the positive characteristics which would enable them to be placed elsewhere. Burkitt's lymphoma is at the upper end of the spectrum, with cell nuclei approximating in size to those of histiocytes, accompanied by a group of histologically similar neoplasms (see below). Convoluted cell lymphoma comprises a separate category and, by definition, the tissue manifestations of the leukaemias are found under this heading, although they are dis-

cussed in detail later (see Chapter 17). This leaves a heterogeneous group of lymphoblastic lymphomas, amongst which are a number showing maturation towards secretory function.

Burkitt's Lymphoma and Lymphomas of Burkitt Type

The entity Burkitt first described occurs predominantly in African children, and has a geographically defined endemic area. The clinical manifestations are well known; a tumour of childhood, rapidly progressive if untreated, and showing a peculiar distribution, with rapidly expanding masses developing outside nodal tissue for the most part. A striking predilection for the jaw bones is apparent in the young age group but multiple tumours of other organs occur. It is known also that there are strong associations between this tumour entity and infection with the Epstein–Barr virus, all of the patients having positive antibody titres.

Sporadic cases with similar clinical features occur in other parts of the world, but in Papua New Guinea, like Africa, the disease is frequent.

The histological appearances of Burkitt's lymphoma are clearly described and illustrated by Berard et al.[6], together with fine points of distinction from similar conditions. The cytological appearance of this tumour is much affected by fixation and this must be borne in mind. At low power, the presence of numerous phagocytic macrophages dispersed amongst the proliferating cells, gives a striking 'starry sky' appearance (Figure 14.3). The background consists of densely packed large lymphoid cells, their round-to-oval nuclei being about the same size as the histiocytic nuclei, with delicately stippled chromatin condensed at the nuclear membrane and occasionally around the few small but distinct nucleoli. This feature can result in the nucleoli appearing as delicate ring-like structures. In histological preparations, the cells seem fairly uniform in size. Depending upon fixation, particularly in formal-saline, the chromatin can appear more clumped and the nucleoli more heavily defined. The narrow rim of cytoplasm is strongly amphophilic and pyroninophilic and may be very sharply defined or imperceptibly blended, again depending upon fixation. The conspicuous lipid vacuoles seen in impression smears are occasionally recognizable in sections. Mitotic figures amongst the lymphoid cells are numerous; the scattered macrophages contain nuclear debris and lipid.

The stage of B lymphocyte development at which Burkitt's lymphoma is engendered remains to be proved. The small non-cleaved follicular centre cell is thought to be the source by some[7, 8] and indeed the appearance is very reminiscent of some florid follicular hyperplasias, especially those seen in childhood. However, no other follicular centre elements are included in the proliferation which characterizes Burkitt's lymphoma.

Other lymphomas are encountered, showing only subtle histological differences from Burkitt's tumour, but in a different clinical setting. They are most frequent in adults, especially in the fifth decade, and predominate in lymph nodes. The patients do not have serum antibodies to the Epstein–Barr virus. The presence of numerous scattered macrophages gives a superficial resemblance to Burkitt's lymphoma, but the cell nuclei are generally a little smaller than those of histiocytes, they vary more in size and outline, not giving such an impression of monotonous, uniform, rounded nuclei. Their chromatin is less delicate, in some cases skein-like and in others more heavily clumped.

To refer to such tumours as lymphoblastic lymphomas of Burkitt type seems appropriate, since it calls to mind an image of densely packed, fairly large lymphoid cells, showing rapid turnover, with numerous interspersed macrophages.

Convoluted Cell Lymphoma

This entity was delineated by Barcos and Lukes[9] and possibly represents neoplastic transformation of T lymphocytes during their stage of development in the thymus. The clinical aspect is of a rapidly growing, extremely radio-sensitive tumour in the mediastinum, most often occurring in young boys, with a rapid progressive course, usually terminating in a leukaemic phase.

In a few cases, study of cell surface markers has indicated that the neoplastic cells are T lymphocytes but, most interestingly, attention has been drawn to the peculiar irregular nuclear outline, summed up in the term convoluted lymphocyte. Admittedly, such a feature is best appreciated in very thin sections, but ordinary histological procedures reveal rather irregular cells, somewhat larger than small lymphocytes, exhibiting numerous mitoses. The amount of cytoplasm is very scanty indeed and the cells tend to appear as naked nuclei (Figure 14.22). A moderate amount of chromatin is present and occasionally a nucleolus can be distinguished. The nuclear convolutions result in deep folds in the nuclear membrane and these produce heavy lines, sometimes in a curious forked arrangement, referred to as a 'chicken's footprint' by Lukes. Cytochemistry shows that these convoluted cells have focal acid phosphatase staining near the nucleus[10], but opinions vary as to whether this is a constant finding.

In a retrospective study of clinically similar cases, Nathwani et al.[11] suggests that the association with convoluted cells is not invariable. Many of their cases were characterized by lymphoid cells indistinguishable from those of acute lymphoblastic leukaemias. However, their study could not include cell marker investigations, and whilst other lymphoblastic lymphomas may present a similar clinical picture, this does not seem to detract from the separate entity of convoluted cell lymphoma, as proposed.

In practice the condition may be encountered when a cervical node is involved, and this may occur before the thymic mass is apparent. The manner in which the cells spread is akin to that of leukaemic infiltrates and they come to displace normal elements of the node without destroying the architecture. Besides recognition of the unusual nuclei, there may be focal PAS positivity, apparently corresponding with the acid phosphatase distribution.

Other 'Lymphoblastic Lymphomas'

It is clear that tissue manifestations of leukaemic disorders, which can precede haematological ab-

normality, occur within this group and these must be considered, particularly in childhood (Figure 17.1). When leukaemia and other distinct entities are excluded, there remains a group of cases having a somewhat variable appearance. Some have a starry-sky pattern due to scattered macrophages, but do not provoke camparison with Burkitt's tumour, since the lymphoid cells are smaller. Others have an undistinguished, sheet-like appearance.

Often a really careful examination, using the oil-immersion objective, coupled with use of the pyronin-methyl-green stain, enables varying degrees of secretory maturation to be recognized, but this is not necessarily associated with abnormalities of serum proteins. There then remains a small number of cases, showing some variation in nuclear and cytoplasmic characteristics, which cannot be diagnosed more precisely on histological grounds alone. They may be designated 'diffuse lymphoma of medium-sized lymphoid cells' or 'lymphoblastic lymphoma', as preference dictates. Such cases are few in practice and merit evaluation with the clinicians concerned, particularly with regard to an unsuspected underlying leukaemic condition.

References

1. Pangalis, G. A., Nathwani, B. N. and Rappaport, H. (1977). Malignant lymphoma, well differentiated lymphocytic. Its relationship with chronic lymphocytic leukaemia and macroglobulinaemia of Waldenström. Cancer, **39**, 999.

2. Harrison, C. V. (1972). The morphology of the lymph node in the macroglobulinaemia of Waldenström. J. Clin. Pathol., **25**, 12.

3. Brunning, R. D. and Parkin, J. (1976). Intranuclear inclusions in plasma cells and lymphocytes from patients with monoclonal gammopathies. Am. J. Clin. Pathol., **66**, 10.

4. Berard, C. W., Jaffe, E. S., Braylan, R. C., Mann, R. B. and Nanba, K. (1978). Immunologic aspects and pathology of the malignant lymphomas. Cancer, **42**, 911.

5. Rappaport, H. (1966). Tumors of the Haematopoietic System. Atlas of Tumor Pathology — Section III — Fascicle 8. (Washington, D.C.: Armed Forces Institute of Pathology).

6. Berard, C. W., O'Conor, G. T., Thomas, L. B. and Torloni, H. (1969). Histopathological definition of Burkitt's tumour. Bull. WHO, **40**, 601.

7. Lukes, R. J. and Collins, R. D. (1975). New approaches to the classification of the lymphomata. Br. J. Cancer, **31** (Suppl. 2), 1.

8. Braylan, R. C., Jaffe, E. S. and Berard, C. W. (1975). Malignant lymphomas: current classification and new observations. In S. C. Sommers (ed.). Hematologic and Lymphoid Pathology. Decennial. 1966–1975, pp. 333–390, (New York: Appleton-Century-Crofts).

9. Barcos, M. P. and Lukes, R. J. (1975). Malignant lymphoma of convoluted lymphocytes. A new entity of possible T-cell type. Progress in Clinical and Biological Research, Vol. 4. Conflicts in Childhood Cancer. L. F. Sinks, and J. O. Godden (eds.), pp. 147–178. (New York: Alan Liss Inc.)

10. Stein, H., Petersen, N., Gaedicke, G., Lennert, K. and Landbeck, G. (1976). Lymphoblastic lymphoma of convoluted or acid phosphatase type — a tumour of T precursor cells. Int. J. Cancer, **17**, 292.

11. Nathwani, B. M., Kim, H. and Rappaport, H. (1976). Malignant lymphoma, lymphoblastic. Cancer, **38**, 964.

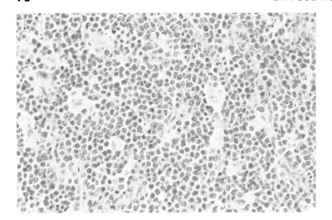

Figure 14.13 African Burkitt's lymphoma. Scattered macrophages impart a 'starry-sky' appearance. H & E ×230.

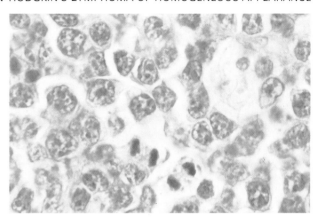

Figure 14.14 African Burkitt's lymphoma. The nuclei of the lymphoid cells tend to be uniform in size, approximating to that of a macrophage included in the field. The chromatin is clumped in pattern and mitoses are frequent. H & E ×910.

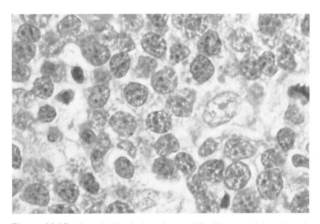

Figure 14.15 Lymphoblastic lymphoma of Burkitt-type. A lymph node from a 54-year-old man had this histological appearance. Epstein–Barr virus antibody titres were negative, bone marrow examination was normal. Before he died two years later, numerous atypical lymphocytes appeared in the peripheral blood. H & E ×910.

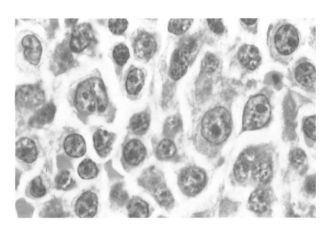

Figure 14.16 A lymphoma of predominantly medium sized cells, although some larger nuclei are included. Definite plasmacytoid differentiation is present, but there was no evidence of an abnormal serum protein. H & E ×910.

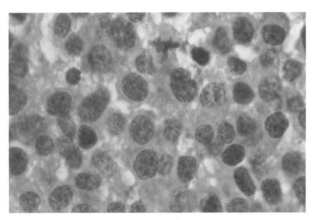

Figure 14.17 A mass in the neck of an elderly man included medium sized lymphoid cells showing definite plasmacytoid differentiation. No abnormality was demonstrable in the serum proteins at the time of presentation and bone marrow examination was unremarkable. H & E ×910.

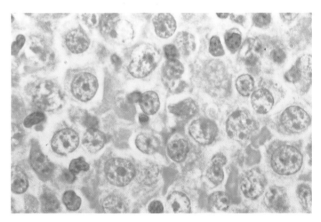

Figure 14.18 A woman of 66 years presented with cervical node enlargement and some obstruction of a para-nasal sinus. The histological appearance of the delicate round nuclei was in favour of lymphoblastic lymphoma, rather than carcinoma. H & E ×910.

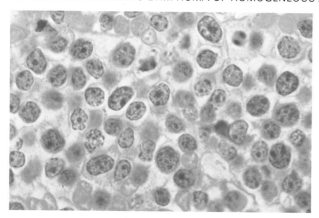

Figure 14.19 Lymphoblastic lymphoma. A middle-aged man complained of malaise and weight loss. An axillary node biopsy consisted of sheets of round to oval cells with delicate nucleoli. Initial bone marrow examination was negative. At necropsy a month later, there was extensive lymphomatous involvement of the gastrointestinal tract. H & E × 910.

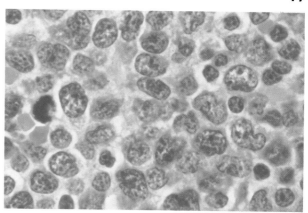

Figure 14.20 Lymphoblastic lymphoma. The cell nuclei of this lymphoma in a middle-aged man show much heavier clumping of the chromatin. This feature is more marked in occasional cells and gives an impression that there is some plasmacytoid differentiation. H & E × 910.

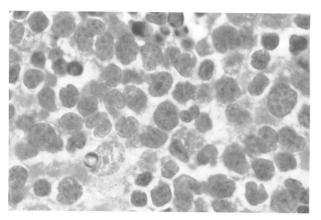

Figure 14.21 Lymphoblastic lymphoma. A man of 67 years presented with a mediastinal mass and generalized lymphadenopathy. A cervical node had this appearance. Many of the medium sized lymphoid cells have a convoluted or folded nuclear outline, but no surface marker studies were performed. H & E × 910.

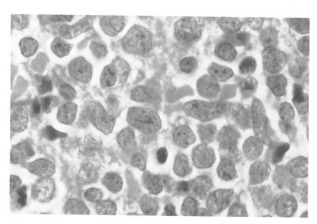

Figure 14.22 An 11-year-old boy presented with a mediastinal mass. Convoluted lymphoid cells, similar to those shown in Figure 14.21, characterized the diffuse lymphoma present. There is no record of a leukaemic phase before his death, one year later. No surface marker studies were performed.

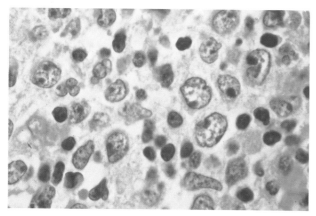

Figure 14.23 Lymphoblastic lymphoma. A woman of 22 years presented with cervical node enlargement and a mass in the upper mediastinum. The neoplastic cells have rather delicate nuclei with a slightly lobulated outline and distinct nucleoli, often near the nuclear membrane. H & E × 910.

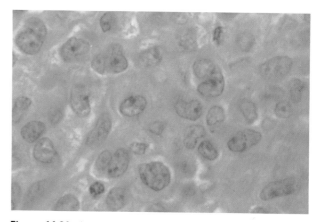

Figure 14.24 Lymphoblastic lymphoma. The cervical node from a 15-year-old girl who also had a mediastinal mass. Allowing for technical differences, the cells resemble those illustrated in Figure 14.23. Although there is a lobulated nuclear outline in both cases, they are clearly different from the nuclei in Figures 14.21 and 14.22, which have prominent folds in their membranes. (These examples demonstrate the limitations of morphology alone in the study of lymphomas). H & E × 910.

Diffuse Non-Hodgkin's Lymphoma of Heterogeneous Appearance

15

Introduction

In the previous section, lymphomas dominated by proliferations of cells predominantly in the same size range are discussed. Attention is drawn, in this section, to those which have a mixed appearance due either to differences in the cytological expression of the basic single cell type or to a conspicuous admixture of other non-neoplastic cells. This group is readily confused with Hodgkin's disease, because of the presence of large nuclei and because of the reactive cell element, especially histiocytes.

Diffuse Lymphoma, Mixed Cell Type

The term 'mixed' in this context refers to cell size; it does not imply origin from more than one cell type, as has been suggested in the past. Although many lymphomas are composed of cells of variable size, this is usually a graduated effect; but in the case in point large and small cells occur, without forms in between, giving the impression of two separate populations. This results from differing forms of the same lymphoid cells, and the diffuse mixed lymphoma is simply the counterpart of lymphomas of obvious follicular pattern, with mixtures of small cleaved and non-cleaved cells (Figures 12.11 and 15.5).

Pleomorphic Histiocytic Lymphoma

This category of unusual neoplasms is referred to by Rappaport[1], and again represents cytological variation in a single cell type. Many of the cells in these cases have features suggestive of histiocytes. They are elongated in shape, with oval nuclei and abundant eosinophilic cytoplasm, which is sometimes rather granular (Figure 15.7). But amongst them are cells with bizarre large nuclei, some of which appear polylobed, and the first impression of such a neoplasm may be that it is a sarcoma. Not surprisingly, this condition is readily confused with lymphocyte depleted Hodgkin's disease.

The features of the large cell nuclei however, are not those of Reed–Sternberg cells. Chromatin staining is heavier overall and the basophilic nucleoli are small, with indistinct margins (Figure 15.8).

Lymphoma of Peripheral T Lymphocytes

Another distinct entity has been described, apparently originating from T lymphocytes within peripheral lymphoid tissue (Mann et al.[2], Waldron et al.[3]). It is a rapidly progressive disease, often accompanied by systemic symptoms, and can occur both in children and adults. Whilst its definitive diagnosis must rest upon cell surface marker studies, nevertheless it has a characteristic histological appearance.

It is composed of lymphoid cells of an extremely mixed appearance (Figure 15·9). Small cells in the infiltrate have irregular nuclear membranes, little cytoplasm and one or two indistinct nucleoli. There are also large cells with vesicular nuclei, sometimes lobulated in form, having prominent eosinophilic nucleoli, with surrounding abundant cytoplasm. Forms intermediate in size and character also occur and collagen bands divide groups of these cells into compartments. The other distinctive feature is the presence of a number of large, acidophil macrophages, which may be in clusters. Jaffe et al.[4] make the interesting suggestion that their presence could be the result of migration inhibition factor, actually produced by the neoplastic T cells.

The diffuse mixed infiltration may obliterate pre-existing nodal tissue but often merely encircles lymphoid follicles, so that a few persist. Vascular proliferation accompanies the cellular expansion; Waldron et al.[3] refer to vessels formed of tall endothelial cells with granular PAS positive cytoplasm. However, other features associated with angio-immunoblastic lymphadenopathy, plasma cells, eosinophils and interstitial acidophilic material are absent.

Lastly, the condition is readily confused with Hodgkin's disease because of the presence of large cells with hyperlobated nuclei and prominent nucleoli, but the pleomorphic nature of the lymphoid infiltrate precludes this diagnosis.

Malignant Lymphoma with a High Content of Epithelioid Histiocytes, Lennert's Lymphoma

This entity has only recently been separated from other lympho-proliferative disorders, and its nature is still enigmatic to some extent. Relatively few cases have so far been described so that the frequency of some clinical features of the condition is still to be assessed.

In 1968, Lennert and Mestdagh[5] drew attention to a group of cases diagnosed as Hodgkin's disease, in which epithelioid histiocytes were numerous and Reed–Sternberg cells were difficult to demonstrate. Although this original group was probably heterogeneous, further studies of cases of this type, including those of Burke and Butler[6] and Kim et al.[7], have suggested that this is an entirely separate entity from Hodgkin's disease, and Lennert himself expressed the same opinion in 1975[8].

Figure 15.1 A diffuse lymphoma composed of a lymphoid element intermixed with clusters of large, pale histiocytes. This cervical node removed from a woman of 66 years was originally interpreted as toxoplasmosis. H & E   × 91.

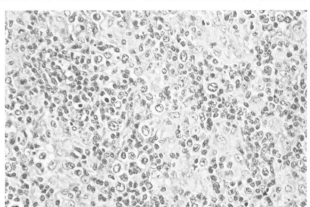

Figure 15.2 Lennert's lymphoma. A lymph node very similar in appearance to that in Figure 15.1. The variation in size of the lymphoid cells is easily appreciated. In 1951 this was thought to be an unusual case of Hodgkin's disease. H & E   × 230.

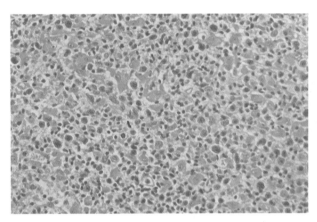

Figure 15.3 An abdominal lymph node from a 69-year-old woman presented this appearance, with abundant eosinophilic histiocytes, not arranged in clusters, amongst lymphoid cells of variable size. See Figure 15.4. H & E   × 230.

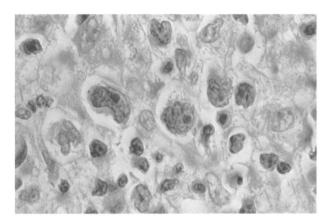

Figure 15.4 Detail of the node shown in Figure 15.3 reveals that the lymphoid cells possess conspicuously convoluted nuclei. Mycosis fungoides was suggested as a possible diagnosis, but there is no evidence of any cutaneous abnormality. However, the nuclear convolution together with the histiocytic infiltration certainly argue for a T cell lymphoma. This case illustrates the limitations of histological appearances alone in the interpretation of lymphomas. H & E   × 910.

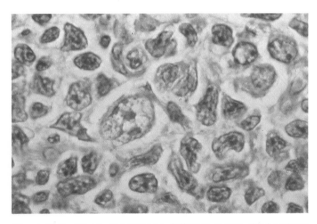

Figure 15.5 Mixed cell lymphoma. Diffuse in pattern, this lymphoma consists of a mixture of smaller cleaved and larger non-cleaved follicular centre cells. H & E   × 910.

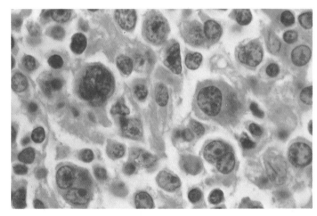

Figure 15.6 Plasma cell tumour. Often these neoplasms show a considerable degree of nuclear pleomorphism, as well as having binucleate forms. H & E   × 910.

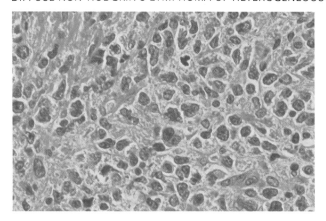

Figure 15.7 Pleomorphic histiocytic lymphoma. An inguinal node from a man of 78 years was replaced by a pleomorphic neoplasm composed of cells with abundant granular eosinophilic cytoplasm. Many of the nuclei are large and bizarre. H & E ×365.

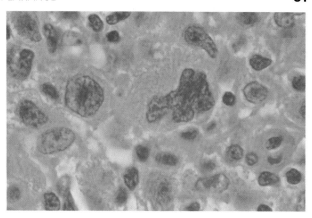

Figure 15.8 Pleomorphic histiocytic lymphoma. A cervical node removed from a woman of 67 years, with generalized lymphadenopathy and hepatomegaly. The general appearance is identical to that in Figure 15.7. The cells with the larger and most bizarre nuclei were focally arranged. H & E ×910.

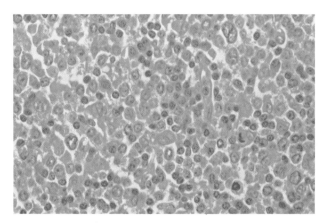

Figure 15.9 Node based T cell lymphoma. A population of lymphoid cells with nuclei of variable size admixed with eosinophilic histiocytes. H & E ×230.

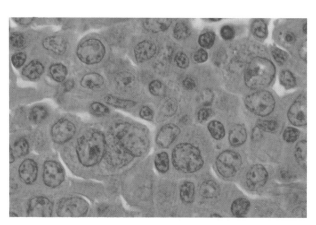

Figure 15.10 Node based T cell lymphoma. Many of the larger lymphoid cells contain a distinctive nucleolus. An occasional nucleus is enlarged and poly-lobed. H & E ×910.
(The author is grateful to Dr R. D. Collins for providing the section illustrated in Figures 15.9 and 15.10).

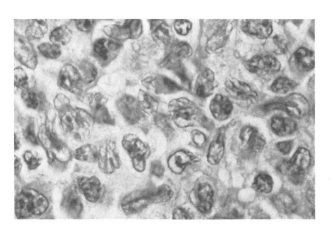

Figure 15.11 Mycosis fungoides. Large cells with vesicular, but excessively convoluted nuclei. H & E ×910.

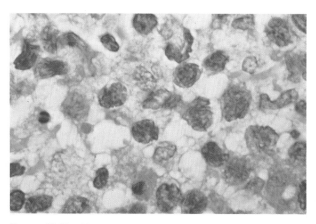

Figure 15.12 Mycosis fungoides. Densely staining, tightly folded nuclei of mycosis cells. H & E ×910.

The majority of patients are in the older age group and present often with already advanced disease, which includes enlargement of the liver and spleen. Involvement of the tonsil occurs, and usually there are systemic symptoms. Despite vigorous therapy, overall survival is short.

Involved lymph nodes show effacement of their architecture, with obliteration of the peripheral sinus and capsular infiltration. Occasional follicles are found to persist amidst the encroaching infiltrate. The most conspicuous feature of the latter is the presence of numerous epithelioid histiocytes, often in clusters, amongst which are proliferating atypical lymphoid cells showing considerable variation in size (Figure 15.2). Larger forms have vesicular nuclei and prominent eosinophilic nucleoli, and the close resemblance to Hodgkin's disease can be well understood. However, it can be firmly excluded by the observation that the accompanying smaller lymphoid cells show atypical features.

Other cells may be included in the infiltrate. Small numbers of eosinophils, neutrophils, plasma cells and multinucleate giant cells of Langhans type occur. Vascular proliferation is not usually a feature but acidophilic, PAS positive intercellular material is deposited.

It is clear that both clinically and histologically there are slight overlaps with angio-immunoblastic lymphadenopathy, but there is no evidence to suggest that the proliferating lymphoid cells are B lymphocytes. and their nature remains to be demonstrated. Two apparent cases of Lennert's lymphoma which evolved further to rather pleomorphic large cell lymphomas are described by Klein et al.[9]. Many of the patients however die of infective causes.

Mycosis Fungoides

In practice, lymph nodes from patients with this primary cutaneous lymphoma are likely to be examined only in the knowledge that there is a pre-existing skin disorder. The difficulty encountered is most likely to be that of recognizing evidence of lymphomatous involvement in nodes already affected by dermatopathic lymphadenopathy.

The dermal infiltrate in mycosis fungoides includes medium-sized lymphoid cells, the nuclei of which are atypical, being dense, slightly elongated and irregular in outline. Two other abnormal cell types contribute to the pleomorphism of the appearance. First, there are those with extremely complex folded nuclei, appeciable even with the light microscope (Figure 15.11), but best demonstrated at ultrastructural level[10] and often referred to as having 'cerebriform' nuclei. Secondly, what have been called 'mycosis' cells, with large and densely staining nuclei which are usually also irregular in outline. It is likely that all the variations are expressions of an underlying neoplastic cell as occurs in other pleomorphic lymphomas. Indeed at necropsy, progression to a much more bizarre, sarcomatous-looking histological picture may have occurred[11].

Positive diagnosis of mycosis fungoides depends therefore on the demonstration of these abnormal cell forms in the lymph nodes. The use of thin sections brings about an increase in the number of positive diagnoses in this disorder, because the dermatopathic background makes interpretation difficult.

Pointers towards lymphomatous involvement are foci of mitotic activity. If these are present, a particularly diligent search for abnormal cells, including re-cutting the blocks at levels, should be undertaken. Although cells with cerebriform nuclei are encountered in the skin in cases of lichen planus[10], their presence in lymph nodes, together with increased mitotic activity undoubtedly indicates a neoplastic disease.

As in all the lymphomas of pleomorphic appearance, mycosis fungoides is readily confused with Hodgkin's disease, not only because some of the large cells resemble Reed–Sternberg cells, but also because the background dermatopathic infiltrate may well include eosinophils and plasma cells as well as numerous histiocytes. Again, in making the distinction, reliance must be placed upon the nature of the lymphocytic infiltrate, and the presence of atypical nuclei excludes the possibility of Hodgkin's disease.

References

1. Rappaport, H. (1966). Tumors of the Hematopoietic System. Atlas of Tumor Pathology — Section III — Fascicle 8. (Washington, D.C.: Armed Forces Institute of Pathology).

2. Mann, R. B., Jaffe, E. S., Braylan, R. C., Eggleston, J. C., Ransom, L., Kaizer, H. and Berard, C. W. (1975). Immunologic and morphologic studies of T cell lymphoma. Am. J. Med., 58, 307.

3. Waldron, J. A., Leech, J. H., Glick, A. D., Flexner, J. M. and Collins, R. D. (1977). Malignant lymphoma of peripheral lymphocyte origin. Cancer, 40, 1604.

4. Jaffe, E. S., Shevach, E. M., Sussman, E. H., Frank, M., Green, I. and Berard, C. W. (1975). Membrane receptor sites for the identification of lymphoreticular cells in benign and malignant conditions. Br. J. Cancer, 31 (Suppl. 2), 107.

5. Lennert, K. and Mestdagh, J. (1968). Lymphogranulomatosen mit Konstant hohem Epitheloidzellgehalt. Virchow's Archiv. Abt. A, 344, 1.

6. Burke, J. S. and Butler, J. J. (1976). Malignant lymphoma with a high content of epithelioid histiocytes (Lennert's lymphoma). Am. J. Clin. Pathol., 66, 1.

7. Kim, H., Jacobs, C., Warnke, R. A., and Dorfman, R. F. (1978). Malignant lymphoma with a high content of epithelioid histiocytes. Cancer, 41, 620.

8. Lennert, K., Mohri, N., Stein, H. and Kaiserling, E. (1975). The histopathology of malignant lymphoma. Br. J. Haemat., 31 (Suppl.), 193.

9. Klein, M. A., Jaffe, R. and Neiman, R. S. (1977). 'Lennert's lymphoma' with transformation to malignant lymphoma, histiocytic type (immunoblastic sarcoma). Am. J. Clin. Pathol., 68, 601.

10. Lutzner, M. A., Hobbs, J. W. and Horvath, P. (1971). Ultrastructure of abnormal cells: in Sezary syndrome, mycosis fungoides and parapsoriasis en plaque. Arch. Derm., 103, 375.

11. Rappaport, H. and Thomas, L. B. (1974). Mycosis fungoides: the pathology of extracutaneous involvement. Cancer, 34, 1198.

16

Histiocytoses

Introduction

Histiocytes play many and varied roles in lymph nodes, providing a passive storage tissue in disposal disorders, increasing in direct response to certain stimuli, or reacting in conjunction with lymphoid cells. They also populate lymphoid tissue where normal components are deficient in either number or function, and thus are found in immune deficiency states, chronic granulomatous disease and cases of congenital rubella[1].

Besides providing the cell of origin for a small number of true histiocytic neoplasms, they often provide a conspicuous element in other lymphomas, either in a frankly phagocytic capacity or in a less easily perceived relationship, possibly under the influence of lymphokines.

But in addition there are other proliferations of histiocytes, systemic in distribution, in which initially at least the process appears to be partially restrained and some degree of function is maintained. These are however progressive conditions, not attributable merely to accumulation of metabolites, and are in the end fatal, although variations in clinical behaviour occur. They comprise the entities known as Letterer–Siwe disease and malignant histiocytosis.

Although the concept of grouping Hand–Schüller–Christian disease and eosinophilic granuloma with Letterer–Siwe disease is an attractive one theoretically, the considerable clinical differences argue for their separation. Cline and Golde[2] link differences in these syndromes with the degree of differentiation of the proliferating histiocytes, and make the point that the chronic disorders may be reactive, rather than neoplastic.

At present, the demonstration of elongated, membrane-bound inclusions within the histiocytes of these proliferative disorders, exactly similar to those first recognized in cutaneous Langerhans cells, is of uncertain significance.

In this account, Hand–Schüller–Christian disease and eosinophilic granuloma have been included with storage disorders, on the basis of the lipid accumulation they may exhibit (see page 34). Perhaps this is inappropriate but it achieves a total separation of these indolent disorders from the progressive and fatal histiocytoses.

Sinus histiocytosis with massive lymphadenopathy has been included in this section because it may be confused by the unwary with malignant histiocytosis. It is however an essentially benign condition in itself, being merely the reflection of an immunological disorder and a viral infection in all probability[3].

Sinus Histiocytosis with Massive Lymphadenopathy

This rare disorder was described in 1969 by Rosai and Dorfman[4], and their study expanded with the addition of further cases in 1972[5]. Although unusual, cases are memorable because of the dramatic histological and clinical appearances associated with them. The majority of reported cases are in patients under twenty years and about half of them are negroes. Almost all have pronounced cervical node enlargement, and often there is some degree of fever. Otherwise they are usually well, but the clinical diagnosis is almost invariably that of lymphoma.

Histologically however, the distinction from lymphoma is clear. Massive sinusoidal dilatation occurs and, although other cells are present, the most conspicuous are large histiocytes, their abundant cytoplasm often foamy and containing apparently intact cells, mainly lymphocytes, but also plasma cells and red cells, (Figure 16.2). Towards the periphery of the node intracytoplasmic nuclei are not seen, but instead, closely packed, apparently replete histiocytes, their cytoplasm bulging with lipid vacuoles and PAS positive material. Often the capsule is thickened and fibrotic, and fibrosis gradually develops in the node itself. Although the lymphoid follicles may be few and small, or entirely absent, the medullary cords are stuffed with plasma cells, often having associated Russell bodies.

The pathogenesis of this peculiar disorder remains obscure but its recognition is important since it appears to run a benign, self-limited course, despite prolonged nodal enlargement.

Letterer–Siwe Disease

Principally a disease of early childhood, the lymph nodes are only involved as part of this systemic disorder. Initially, histiocytes distend the sinuses and are easily recognizable as such, with oval or slightly indented nuclei and eosinophilic cytoplasm which may contain lipid vacuoles and show some evidence of phagocytosis. Later there is spread into the deep cortex and finally crowding out of the follicles. In the earlier stages, a few multinucleated cells may be seen; later the cells have a less differentiated appearance. The number of eosinophil leukocytes appearing in the infiltrate is variable, and they may be very few in some cases.

Malignant Histiocytosis

This condition was described by Scott and Robb-Smith in 1939[6], using the term 'histiocytic medul-

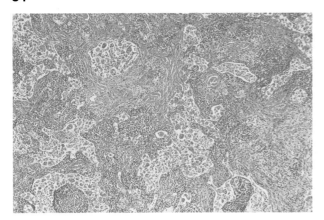

Figure 16.1 Sinus histiocytosis with massive lymphadenopathy. Cellular cords separate the widely dilated sinuses. There is evidence of gradual fibrosis. H & E ×36.5.

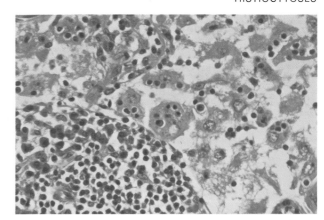

Figure 16.2 Sinus histiocytosis with massive lymphadenopathy. Plasma cells are seen to be numerous in the cord adjoining the sinus; numerous enlarged histiocytes present contain multiple muclei within their cytoplasm. H & E ×230.

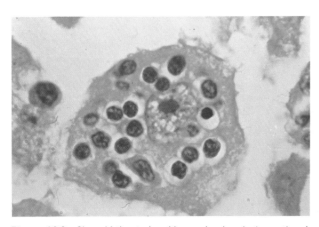

Figure 16.3 Sinus histiocytosis with massive lymphadenopathy. A single enlarged histiocyte containing apparently intact nucleated cells. H & E ×910.

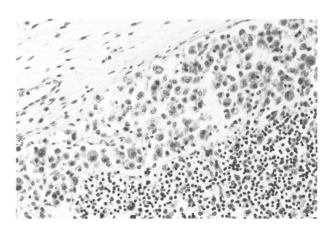

Figure 16.4 Malignant histiocytosis. A 16-year-old boy who died only six weeks after the onset of his illness. The subcapsular sinus of a lymph node obtained at necropsy shows numerous histiocytes, unremarkable in appearance, except for conspicuous erythrophagocytosis. H & E ×230.

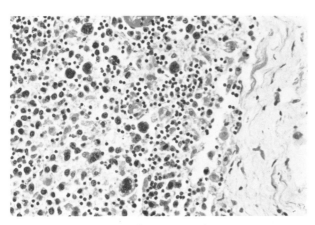

Figure 16.5 (from the same case as Figure 16.4). Elsewhere in the lymph nodes, the pleomorphic nature of the histiocytes is clearly demonstrated. H & E ×230.

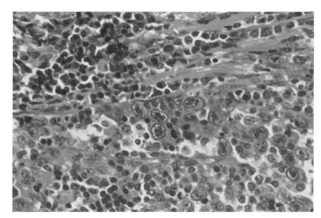

Figure 16.6 Malignant histiocytosis. Death followed 4 weeks after this enlarged inguinal node was removed from a man of 46 years. The bizarre nature of the cells which distend all the sinuses, together with lack of evidence of erythrophagocytosis, led to difficulty with the initial diagnosis, but the necropsy findings were those of malignant histiocytosis. H & E ×365.

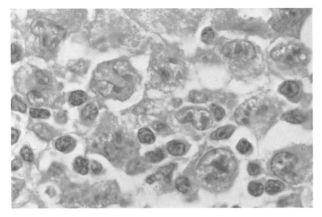

Figure 16.7 Malignant histiocytosis. A case in which, whilst still recognizably histiocytes, the proliferating cells are clearly abnormal. H & E ×910.

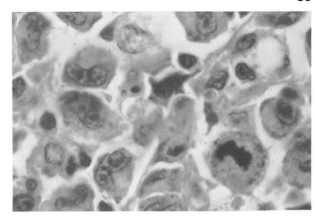

Figure 16.8 Malignant histiocytosis. An axillary node from a man of 29 years. Resemblance to normal histiocytes is only poorly maintained, but erythrophagocytosis is a helpful diagnostic feature. H & E ×910.

lary reticulosis'. Patients present with fever and weight loss; commonly they have generalized lymph node enlargement, together with involvement of liver and spleen. Males predominate over females by at least two to one and although the disorder can occur at any age, the majority are under forty years, with a not insignificant number of cases in the first decade.

Often already ill at the time of presentation, the disease progresses rapidly with reduction in all cellular elements in the blood and often a preterminal phase of jaundice. Despite vigorous chemotherapy, the mean survival is little more than a year, although occasional long term remissions have occurred[7]. Vardiman et al.[8] reported four unusual cases whose first symptom was due to splenomegaly, and have suggested that there may be a more chronic form of the condition. In view of the behaviour of histiocytic proliferations in general, this would not be surprising.

The essential feature of the lymph nodes in this condition is the proliferation of histiocytes within the sinuses, sometimes most marked in the sub-capsular sinus (Figure 16.4), and contrasting therefore with the common reactive sinus histiocytosis. The extent to which the histiocytes differ from normal is tremendously variable. Often, the individual cells show no atypical features, but there may be considerable erythrophagocytosis. On the other hand, phagocytic activity can be almost absent, and it may be difficult to recognize the pleomorphic cells with amphophilic cytoplasm as histiocytes, the appearance closely resembling infiltration of the sinuses by an anaplastic carcinoma (Figure 16.6).

In either case, invasion of the node pulp itself can occur, although this may well take place earlier in what appear to be more aggressive forms of the disease. At necropsy, examination of lymph nodes from differing sites may reveal all grades of 'differentiation' and invasion. In some areas, banal histiocytes are noticeable chiefly by increase in their numbers, whilst elsewhere large and bizarre cells invade the node pulp, frequently accompanied by haemorrhage. Wolfson et al.[9],

reported a case with features similar to malignant histiocytosis, but multinucleated giant cells formed a conspicuous element in the histiocytic proliferation.

A group of rare disorders is encountered in babies and very young children, often referred to as familial haemophagocytic reticuloses[10, 11]. These cases occur in siblings and have also been noted in more than one generation. The histological appearance is entirely akin to that of malignant histiocytosis, but whether the relationship has any other definite parallels, remains to be shown.

References

1. Claman, H. N., Suvatte, V., Githens, J. H. and Hathaway, W. E. (1970). Histiocytic reaction in dysgammaglobulinaemia and congenital rubella. Paediatrics, **46**, 89.

2. Cline, M. J. and Golde, D. W. (1973). A review and re-evaluation of the histiocytic disorders. Am. J. Med., **55**, 49.

3. Lober, M., Rawlings, W., Newell, G. R. and Reed, R. J. (1973). Sinus histiocytosis with massive lymphadenopathy. Report of a case associated with elevated EBV antibody titers. Cancer, **32**, 421.

4. Rosai, J. and Dorfman, R. F. (1969). Sinus histiocytosis with massive lymphadenopathy. Arch. Pathol., **87**, 63.

5. Rosai, J. and Dorfman, R. F. (1972). Sinus histiocytosis with massive lymphadenopathy: a pseudolymphomatous benign disorder. Cancer, **30**, 1174.

6. Scott, R. B. and Robb-Smith, A. H. T. (1939). Histiocytic medullary reticulosis. Lancet, **2**, 194.

7. Warnke, R. A., Kim, H. and Dorfman, R. F. (1975). Malignant histiocytosis (histiocytic medullary reticulosis). Cancer, **35**, 215.

8. Vardiman, J. W., Byrne, G. E. and Rappaport, H. (1975). Malignant histiocytosis with massive splenomegaly in asymptomatic patients. A possible chronic form of the disease. Cancer, **36**, 419.

9. Wolfson, W. L., Gossett, T. and Pagani, J. (1976). Systemic giant-cell histiocytosis. Cancer, **38**, 2529.

10. Farquhar, J. W. and Claireaux, A. E. (1952). Familial haemophagocytic reticulosis. Arch. Dis. Childh. **27**, 519.

11. Bell, R. J. M., Brafield, A. J. E., Barnes, N. D. and France, N. E. (1968). Familial haemophagocytic reticulosis. Arch. Dis. Childh., **43**, 601.

Chronic Lymphocytic Leukaemia

The appearance of the lymph nodes is identical to that seen in lymphocytic lymphoma[1] (Chapter 14). Normal functional compartments are over-run by small lymphocytes, and amongst these appear to a greater or lesser degree, foci of larger and less mature lymphoid cells, similar to those seen in the blood and bone marrow in chronic lymphocytic leukaemia.

These have round to oval, open nuclei and distinct nucleoli. Some have the features of pro-lymphocytes, others of blast cells. These focal areas have been referred to as proliferation centres or pseudonodules[2] (Figure 17.7). Sometimes they are sufficiently accentuated to cause possible confusion with follicular lymphomas, but a reticulin stain fails to show a true underlying nodular growth pattern. In the rare prolymphocytic leu-kaemias, more of the immature cells appear in the lymph nodes. Rarely, there is a change to a much more primitive cytological appearance, referred to and illustrated by Dick and Maca[3], so that cells they refer to as pleomorphic blast cells can cause confusion with Hodgkin's disease and other lymphomas.

The majority of cases of chronic lymphocytic leukaemia represent proliferations of B lymphocytes, which are able to leave the bone marrow and popu-late lymph nodes. The only difference between this condition and lymphocytic lymphoma is presumably that the neoplastic transformation occurs at a slightly later stage of development in the latter case, and therefore initially the prime proliferative site is within the lymph nodes themselves, rather than the bone marrow.

Acute Lymphoblastic Leukaemia

Enlarged lymph nodes are a frequent accompaniment of this disease, and they are infiltrated by the almost round, rather fragile immature lymphoid cells, similar to the lymphoblasts present in the bone marrow. Where the condition is not suspected initially, this appearance may at first be classified as a diffuse non-Hodgkin's lymphoma of medium-sized cells, or 'lymphoblastic' type. In this case at least, the term 'lymphoblastic' is entirely appropriate. It has already been stressed that, whenever a neoplastic proliferation in this general category is encountered, the possibility of an underlying leukaemia should be considered.

Even when no abnormalities have been reported in the peripheral blood, it is essential to examine the bone marrow. Before the overt stage of acute lymphoblastic leukaemia develops, it is possible to have an involved lymph node or the development of soft tissue masses, especially in young children. In view of the prognostic and therapeutic impli-cations, early diagnosis is important and should be suggested by the monotonous appearance of the infiltrate of uniform, round, blast-like cells with numerous mitotic figures, and by the ease with which they distort prior to fixation.

There are also rare cases of granulocytic leukaemia in which, when blastic crisis occurs, the blast cells are found to have features more re-sembling lymphoblasts and in fact the patients respond best to a treatment regimen designed for acute lymphoblastic leukaemia. This alteration in their disease may be accompanied by enlargement of the lymph nodes which, if biopsied, have a histological appearance indistinguishable from that of acute lymphoblastic leukaemia.

Granulocytic Leukaemias

The nodal sinuses contain leukaemic cells which, whilst easily recognized in chronic myeloid leu-kaemia, are not so obvious in acute forms of the disease. Usually the presence of an occasional cell with pronounced eosinophil cytoplasmic granules indicates the nature of the abnormal cells. Later, the process invades the node and it may not be possible to appreciate that the infiltrate emanates from the sinuses.

Extra-nodal soft tissue masses formed of primi-tive myeloid cells can develop, similar to the phenomenon which occurs in acute lymphoblastic leukaemia. Formerly known as chloromas, because of the greenish hue of the cut surfaces, they are now termed 'granulocytic sarcomas'. These curious masses can appear prior to other manifestations of the leukaemia[4] and they then generate con-siderable diagnostic problems, since it is not easy to recognize primitive myeloid cells out of their usual milieu and prepared by histological tech-niques. They appear as fairly large cells with oval nuclei, sometimes a little indented, containing a moderate amount of stippled chromatin and oc-casionally a distinct nucleolus. Their cytoplasm is eosinophilic, slightly granular and ill-defined (Figure 17.2). Most commonly they are confused with histiocytes, but the nuclei are really too rounded, and too large, relative to the cell, for histiocytes. Mitoses may be numerous.

A detailed examination using the oil immersion lens should enable cells with eosinophil granules to be recognized. To confirm the diagnosis, the naphthol AS-D chloroacetate esterase reaction should be positive.

Leukaemic cells can demonstrate phagocytic

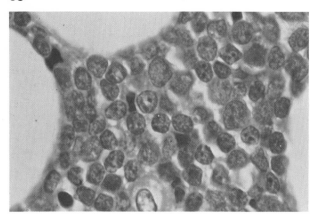

Figure 17.1 A six-month-old boy presented with an enlarged post-auricular lymph node. This was replaced by almost round lymphoid cells, having moderately dense nuclear chromatin and little cytoplasm. These cells extended freely into adjacent soft tissue. A few months later, frank leukaemia developed. Acute lymphoblastic leukaemia. H & E   ×910.

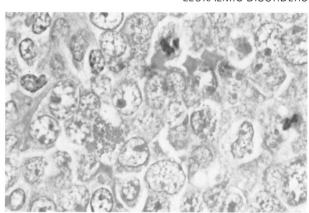

Figure 17.2 Acute myeloid leukaemia. An enlarged node removed from a patient already known to have this condition shows replacement by large blast-like cells, some of which have large eosinophilic cytoplasmic granules. H & E   ×910.

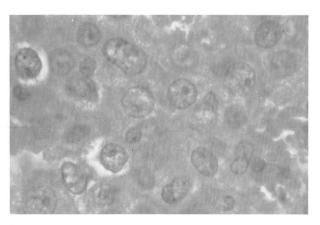

Figure 17.3 Granulocytic sarcoma. A man of 46 years presented with a mass in the soft tissues of the upper thigh. Eosinophil precursors were not readily seen in the H & E stained section but an esterase stain was positive. H & E   ×910.

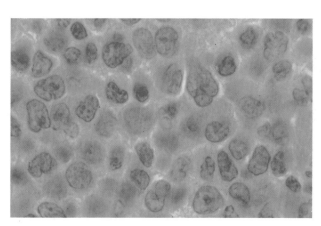

Figure 17.4 A man of 38 years presented with fever and generalized lymphadenopathy. The peripheral blood examination showed no abnormality. A cervical node biopsy had this appearance. Despite the unusual nature of the cell nuclei, occasional cells with eosinophil cytoplasmic granules led to the diagnosis of myeloid leukaemia. Subsequent bone marrow examination revealed atypical myelo-monocytic leukaemia. H & E   ×910.

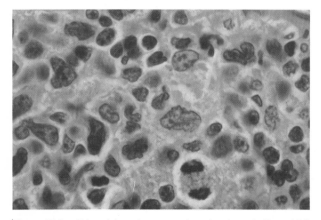

Figure 17.5 Although from the same node as that shown in Figure 17.4, this tissue was not fixed in formal-saline, but in a fixative which included mercuric chloride. The difference in the cytological appearance is considerable. H & E   ×910.

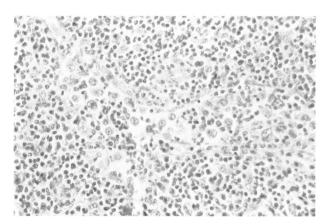

Figure 17.6 In more chronic forms of myeloid leukaemias, the picture is that of abnormal cells mainly within the sinuses, with minimum invasion of the nodal pulp. H & E   ×230.

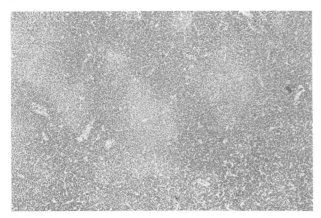

Figure 17.7 Chronic lymphocytic leukaemia. Paler proliferation centres are apparent upon low power examination. In other cases, the appearance may be that of a uniform sheet of unremarkable small lymphocytes. H & E ×36.5.

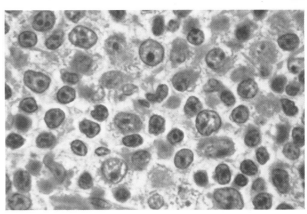

Figure 17.8 Chronic lymphocytic leukaemia. Foci of larger lymphoid cells, resembling those seen in the bone marrow, contribute to the differing appearance of the proliferation centres. H & E ×910.

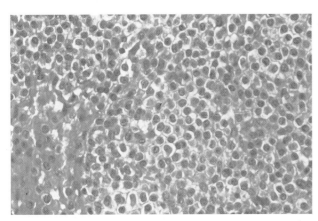

Figure 17.9 Hairy cell leukaemia. The monotonous appearance of the cells at low power is shown. In this example a shrinkage artefact makes each nucleus appear surrounded by a clear halo. H & E ×365.

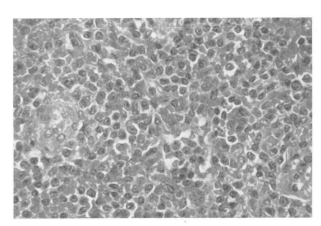

Figure 17.10 Hairy cell leukaemia. Cells in the spleen from the same case as Figure 17.9. Again, a monotonous appearance, but the appearance of oval nuclei, surrounded by discernible cytoplasm is more characteristic. H & E ×365.

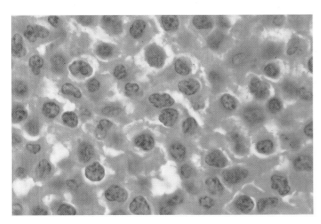

Figure 17.11 Hairy cell leukaemia. At high power, some irregularity of the nuclei is appreciable. H & E ×910.

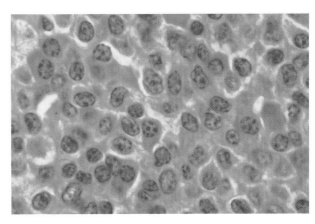

Figure 17.12 Hairy cell leukaemia. Areas of a very intimate relationship with obvious plasma cells can be found readily in some cases. H & E ×910.

activity and in cases of myelo-monocytic leukaemia, there can be prominent erythrophagocytosis by large cells within sinuses. Clearly this change, in the absence of other evidence, could be misinterpreted as malignant histiocytosis (Chapter 16).

In post-mortem material particularly, it is often very difficult to differentiate the two conditions, acute leukaemia and malignant histiocytosis, considering H & E sections of the lymph nodes alone. A careful evaluation of the infiltrate in other organs is required, together with histochemistry.

Leukaemic Reticulo-endotheliosis, 'Hairy Cell' Leukaemia

The clinical features of this condition are by now well recognized[5, 6], but it can still present occasionally as a diagnostic problem to the histopathologist. Often an enlarged node is submitted in conjunction with the spleen, since the cellular proliferation is pre-eminent in that organ.

In lymph nodes, the process of infiltration spreads from the sinuses, to isolate the lymphoid follicles first and then to replace the entire node. The most striking feature of the infiltrate is appreciated at medium power examination and this is its monotony (Figure 17.9). It is related to the overall uniformity in size of the cells, although high power examination reveals that there is a little variation.

The nuclei tend to be oval, their length being approximately 1½ times the diameter of a normal small lymphocyte nucleus. Their chromatin is much less dense than that of normal lymphocytes, but quite well-defined clumps are present, together with lines, which may be folds in the nuclear membrane. There are no distinct nucleoli. Occasional larger, slightly irregular and denser nuclei are seen and rarely, tiny clusters of cells whose nuclei appear almost convoluted (Figure 17.11). Mitotic figures are virtually absent. The cells have a moderate amount of cytoplasm and, depending upon fixation, this can appear as a clear halo surrounding the nucleus, or palely eosinophilic with either a homogeneous texture or slightly granular appearance. In histological preparations, usually there is no evidence of the curious, long, thin cytoplasmic processes which give rise to the name 'hairy cell' leukaemia. But occasionally, when the cells are suspended in fluid, as in a sinus, then a delicate fringed cytoplasmic margin can be seen.

The precise nature of these 'hairy cells' remains uncertain, since features of both macrophage/monocyte behaviour and surface characteristics of B lymphocytes have been reported[7]. In two of the cases investigated, the presence of persistent surface Ig of a single light chain type was found, and occasional cases associated with serum paraproteins occur. There is no doubt that recognizable mature plasma cells are to be observed intimately mixed with the hairy cells in some cases (Figure 17.12), and can even be associated with scattered clumps of Russell bodies. The significance of observations such as this remain to be assessed since they could just as well represent an associated reactive component, rather than an integral one.

When the diagnosis is under consideration, and histo- or cytochemical techniques are available, then the cells can be assessed for the presence of tartrate resistant acid phosphatase[8], since possession of this iso-enzyme is considered to be almost specific for hairy cells.

References

1. Lukes, R. J. and Collins, R. D. (1975). New approaches to the classification of the lymphomata. Br. J. Cancer, **31** (Suppl. 2), 1.
2. Dick, F. R. (1977). Pseudonodular and mixed lymphocytic patterns in the lymph node of chronic lymphocytic leukaemia patients. Am. J. Clin. Pathol., **67**, 210. (Abstract).
3. Dick, F. R. and Maca, R. D. (1978). The lymph node in chronic lymphocytic leukaemia. Cancer, **41**, 283.
4. Mason, T. E., Demaree, R. S. Jr., and Margolis, C. I. (1973). Granulocytic sarcoma (chloroma) two years preceding myelogenous leukaemia. Cancer, **31**, 423.
5. Burke, J. S., Byrne, G. E. Jr. and Rappaport, H. (1974). Hairy cell leukaemia (leukaemic reticuloendotheliosis). I. A clinical pathologic study of 21 patients. Cancer, **33**, 1399.
6. Katayama, I. and Finkel, H. E. (1974). Leukaemic reticuloendotheliosis. A clinicopathologic study with review of the literature. Am. J. Med., **57**, 115.
7. Braylan, R. C., Jaffe, E. S., Triche, T. J., Nanba, K., Fowlkes, B. J., Metzger, H., Frank, M. M., Dolan, M. S., Yee, C. L., Green, I. and Berard, C. W. (1978). Structural and functional properties of the 'hairy' cells of leukaemic reticuloendotheliosis. Cancer, **41**, 210.
8. Yam, L. T., Li, C. Y. and Finkel, H. E. (1972). Leukaemic reticuloendotheliosis. The role of tartrate resistant acid phosphatase in diagnosis and splenectomy in treatment. Arch. Int. Med., **130**, 248.

Introduction

Reference to problems in diagnosis has already been made, but in this section a few further difficult areas are mentioned, particularly those where different conditions show some overlap in their histological appearances.

Proliferations having a Nodular Configuration

In a number of conditions, the initial low-power examination gives an impression that all normal features have been replaced by cellular tissue arranged in focal aggregates. These may show a variable degree of resemblance to normal follicles and their centres, being complete of course in follicular hyperplasia, which in extreme cases may dominate the entire node. The underlying nodularity is accentuated by use of a reticulin stain, with an exception in the case of the 'pseudofollicles' which can occur in both chronic lymphocytic leukaemia and lymphocytic lymphoma. The paler proliferation centres which can be so striking are often not discernible in the reticulin preparation, but may occasionally be recognized as areas deficient in fibres.

In Hodgkin's disease, there can be well-marked nodularity in the lymphocyte predominant form, quite apart from the sub-type which is entitled 'nodular'. Amongst the non-Hodgkin's group, the follicular lymphomas are the most frequent and can usually be recognized on the basis of cytological uniformity and habit of follicular formation, even where invading adipose tissue, either in the centre of the node itself or outside it. However, in a very small number of cases, it is not possible to distinguish the very earliest phases of follicular lymphoma with confidence. It may be suspected, but not certain. A report on such cases should be worded with care. If the condition is indeed a lymphoma usually another node enlarges within a few months and definite diagnostic features are then present. It is wiser to withhold treatment until this occurs since other patients, with entirely similar biopsy appearances, have subsequently remained asymptomatic for several years.

Where the histological appearance suggests half-formed follicular structures, with layers of small lymphocytes wrapped around pale centres, this is characteristic of angiofollicular hyperplasia (Figures 18.1, 10.3), but occasionally a suggestion of rather less organized follicular structures can be seen in immunoblastic lymphadenopathy (Figure 18.3).

Lastly, the problems attached to assessing nodular proliferations which vaguely resemble Hodgkin's disease are discussed at the end of Chapter 11.

Increase in Histiocytes in a Lymph-Node

In any investigation, the appropriate questions must be asked, and this seems especially relevant in the present context. Most of these questions should be answered during the initial low-power examination. The plurality of roles played by cells of the monocyte/macrophage type has been referred to already, and where they appear in increased numbers it is essential to try to understand what emphasis in their normal behaviour this represents.

First, is their presence particularly related to any of the functional compartments? Can it be explained by any exogenous material or micro-organisms or, alternatively, is there excess of some endogenous product? Do they exhibit granulomatous behaviour, as part of either a normal or abnormal immunological response? Does the increase appear to be compensatory, because of lack of some other normal component, for instance, granular phagocytes? Do the histiocytes accompany a neoplastic proliferation of some other cell type, either in a straightforward phagocytic capacity or in some more complex relationship? Lastly, could they represent a true neoplasm arising from the histiocytes themselves? If this is under consideration as a possibility, it is well to remember that such neoplasms are rare, and to consider whether the cells in question are truly histiocytic. Some epithelial neoplasms include oval cells, whose nuclei resemble those of histiocytes (Figure 18.12).

Increased Histiocytes in Association with Eosinophils

In many situations, histiocytes are accompanied by eosinophils, which no doubt reflects some normal function. The reason for making special mention of this is that the presence of eosinophils within infiltrates predisposes to the diagnosis of Hodgkin's disease, and may be used as the final argument in a case which is difficult to resolve. Such an assertion loses its force if it is realized that the role eosinophils play in Hodgkin's disease is probably no different from their role in many other situations, and their presence is no more an indication of a specific lymphoma than is the presence of any other inflammatory cell.

Some of the other conditions in which eosinophils occur, and may be numerous, are dermatopathic lymphadenopathy, drug induced reactions, allergic granulomatosis, immunoblastic lymphadenopathy

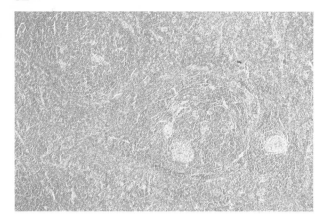

Figure 18.1 A nodular proliferation in which thick walled blood vessels can be distinguished and a semblance of arrangement of lymphocytes in concentric rings about a central focus. Angiofollicular hyperplasia. H & E ×36.5.

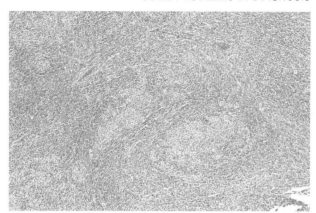

Figure 18.2 A similar appearance to that seen in Figure 18.1 but the central part of the nodular areas contains many large, abnormal cells. This was thought most likely to represent early Hodgkin's disease, but no diagnostic Reed-Sternberg cells were demonstrable. H & E ×36.5.

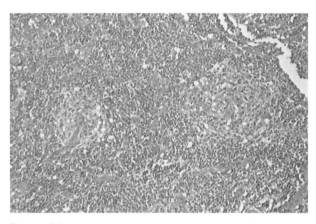

Figure 18.3 The presence of pseudofollicular structures in a case of angioimmunoblastic lymphadenopathy also gives a nodular pattern. H & E ×36.5.

Figure 18.4 The rather poorly preserved cervical lymph node, from a woman of 77 years, shows a definite nodular pattern in some areas but elsewhere the proliferation was diffuse. (See Figure 18.5 from the same case). H & E ×36.5.

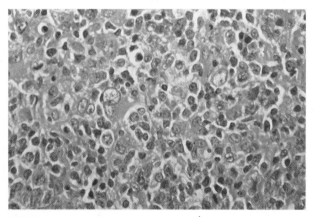

Figure 18.5 The cell population is composed of lymphoid cells of variable size and appearance, admixed with large phagocytic histiocytes (in places much more numerous than shown here) and scattered eosinophils. Occasional much larger cells present had distinct nucleoli. Cytologically at least, this case comes closest to Lennert's lymphoma, although the nodularity is not typical. H & E ×365.

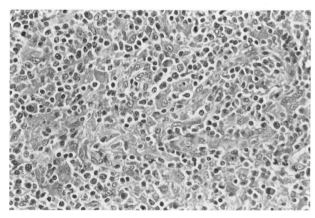

Figure 18.6 Normal lymphoid tissue is replaced by thick walled blood vessels lying amongst lymphocytes, plasma cells and large, eosinophilic histiocytes. There was no intercellular PAS-positive material but the serum contained a slight increase of gammaglobulins. Probably this is a form of angioimmunoblastic lymphadenopathy. It could be confused with Lennert's lymphoma. H & E ×230.

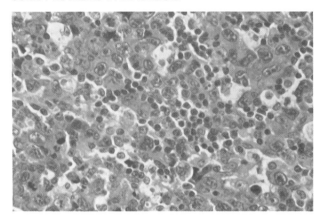

Figure 18.7 The sinuses of this inguinal node were distended by darkly staining pleomorphic cells. It was suggested that the patient might have a malignant teratoma of the testis, but the condition proved to be malignant histiocytosis (see also Figure 16.5). H & E ×365.

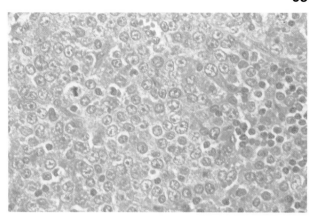

Figure 18.8 An occasional cell with eosinophilic cytoplasmic granules was noted in this large cell population. The naphthol AS-D chloroacetate esterase reaction was positive. Granulocytic sarcoma. H & E ×365.

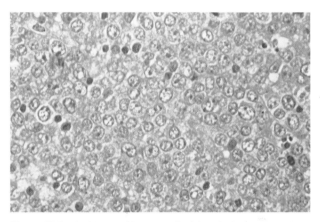

Figure 18.9 A 61-year-old woman had lymphadenopathy, spleno-megaly, pyrexia and a pericardial effusion. This node was interpreted as undifferentiated carcinoma but the delicate round nuclei of the cells, together with lack of cohesive growth, are more consistent with the clinical impression of lymphoma. Bone marrow examination was negative. H & E ×365.

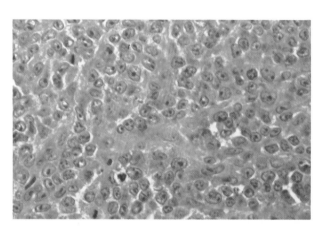

Figure 18.10 A cervical node from a middle-aged man contains oval cells which include frequent mitotic figures and show a semblance of arrangement. A poorly differentiated carcinoma. H & E ×365.

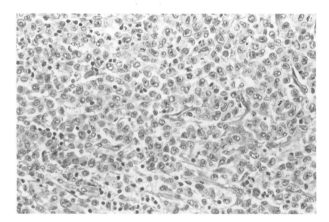

Figure 18.11 A woman of 44 years presented initially with some lymph node enlargement and was thought to have a histiocytic lymphoma. However, there is a tendency for the rather uniform and neat cells to be arranged in swathes and in places they appeared cohesive. (See Figure 18.12 from the same case). H & E ×230.

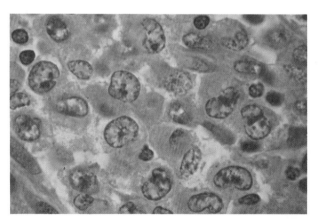

Figure 18.12 Occasional kidney-shaped nuclei are reminiscent of histiocytes and there is a moderate amount of eosinophilic cytoplasm associated with the cells. However at subsequent necropsy, the wide-spread neoplasm was felt to be more consistent with a carcinoma, although the primary site was uncertain. H & E ×910.

and Lennert's lymphoma as well as other pro-liferations which are primarily histiocytic.

Increase in Cells within Sinuses

Although the common sinus histiocytosis contri-butes to the changes found in many conditions, in some cases it is an increase in the population of cells within sinuses which dominates the histo-logical appearance, or at least makes a significant contribution. The population in question may be a uniform one, or have a pleomorphic appearance. It may either appear to derive from sinus histiocytes themselves, or perhaps suggest an origin from elsewhere.

Although usually accompanied by other charac-teristic changes in any particular case, the alto-gether striking appearance of densely packed, extremely uniform oval cells of 'immature' or 'unripe' sinus histiocytosis should be mentioned (Figure 8.2). This is characteristic of toxoplasmosis, but occurs also in brucellosis and other conditions. It contrasts with common forms of histiocytosis where the cells are much more variable in ap-pearance.

If, in a node showing sinus histiocytosis, the condition is just as marked, or even more con-spicuous, in the outer part of the node and there is also evidence of erythrophagocytosis, no matter how benign the proliferation appears at first sight the possibility of malignant histiocytosis must be borne in mind. The degree of nuclear abnormality and cellular pleomorphism is extremely variable in malignant histiocytosis (see page 85), but a detailed search may result in the finding of an occasional, rather large, hyperchromatic nucleus.

Although the histiocytic accumulations in storage disorders begin within the sinuses, they rapidly in-vade the pulp of the node itself, and often include multinucleate giant cells and some eosinophils.

The presence of enormous histiocytes within the sinuses, often containing the nuclei of other cells within their cytoplasm, is indicative of the extra-ordinary and rare condition of sinus histiocytosis with massive lymphadenopathy (see page 83) This is so unusual in appearance that it is unlikely to be confused with anything else.

The assessment of a pleomorphic population within sinuses can be difficult, because on the one hand this can be a manifestation of malignant histiocytosis (Figure 18.7), and on the other may represent invasion by a non-lymphoid tumour, such as a malignant melanoma or an extremely poorly differentiated carcinoma. Only a detailed search may reveal small areas where the cells seem to be separate from one another and to resemble histiocytes. Convincing evidence of erythrophago-cytosis may be scanty or even lacking. But even in such an undifferentiated form of malignant histiocytosis, striking sinus distribution may be maintained, contrasting with sheet-like areas of

carcinomas, which readily invade the adjacent nodal tissue.

Other conditions giving rise to abnormal cells within sinuses include extra-medullary haemo-poiesis, usually recognized because of the presence of megakaryocytes, non-lymphoid leukaemic in-filtration, and occasionally lymphoma cells them-selves, spreading via the lymphatics (Figure 12.12).

Diffuse Sheets of Large Uniform Cells replacing Normal Architecture

In such cases, it is not always possible to distinguish between a large cell lymphoma and a very poorly differentiated carcinoma. In the region of the nasopharynx in particular, almost undifferentiated carcinomas arise, lacking in pattern altogether. The nuclear characteristics may be recognized as atypical for any of the lymphomas, but even this may be equivocal. The tendency for epithelial neoplastic cells to adhere to one another often results in some semblance of arrangement of the cells, with the formation of 'nests' or compartments. However, certain of the large cell lymphomas show similar compartmentalization, by intervening re-ticulin fibres, so this cannot be regarded as an entirely reliable diagnostic feature. Rather, one has to form an impression of whether or not the cells seem cohesive and grow as sheets, rather than quite separate from one another.

Even where the cells are less primitive in appearance, perhaps somewhat resembling histio-cytes, being more elongated, with oval nuclei, distinction between a histiocytic lymphoma and carcinoma can still be difficult. But in general terms, the carcinoma may tend to have a 'neater' appearance, due to more uniformity of nuclear size and shape, and may betray a semblance of cells arranged in broad swathes (Figure 18.11).

A histiocytic lymphoma may also be readily confused with the rare neoplasm composed almost exclusively of large cleaved follicular centre cells (Figure 13.7). The nuclei of the latter however tend to be more angulated, perhaps with obvious notches, apparent folds in the nuclear membrane and only small, indistinct nucleoli, where visible. This contrasts with the somewhat humped outline of the nuclei of neoplastic histiocytes, which often tend to be vesicular and contain a well-defined nucleolus (Figure 14.9). Usually also their cyto-plasm is abundant and obviously eosinophilic, whereas that of cleaved cells is frequently difficult to appreciate at all, and appears to shrink, leaving only a clear space.

Before appending the final diagnosis of histio-cytic lymphoma, an effort should be made to identify any residual sinuses and to find evidence of erythrophagocytosis (Figure 16.8), in case the underlying disorder is really that of malignant histiocytosis.

Index